Neurological Problems in the Elderly - Bridging Current State and New Outlooks

Edited by Patricia Bozzetto Ambrosi

Published in London, United Kingdom

Neurological Problems in the Elderly - Bridging Current State and New Outlooks
http://dx.doi.org/10.5772/intechopen.1004686
Edited by Patricia Bozzetto Ambrosi

Contributors
Brink M. Ntjana, Caroline Bozzetto Ambrosi, Chenelle Ribeiro-Wagener, Elena Shanina, Firdevs Ezgi Uçan Tokuç, Patricia Bozzetto Ambrosi, Priya Dey, Qiyi Yu, Robert Glenn Smith, Terry Jeremy Ellapen, Vishal Singh, Xianda Ma, Yidong Zhang, Yifan Wu, Yuxiao Chen, Yvonne Paul

First published in London, United Kingdom, 2025 by IntechOpen
IntechOpen is the global imprint of INTECHOPEN LIMITED, registered in England and Wales, registration number: 11086078, 167-169 Great Portland Street, London, W1W 5PF, United Kingdom

For EU product safety concerns: IN TECH d.o.o., Prolaz Marije Krucifikse Kozulić 3, 51000 Rijeka, Croatia, info@intechopen.com or visit our website at intechopen.com.

British Library Cataloguing-in-Publication Data
A catalogue record for this book is available from the British Library

Neurological Problems in the Elderly - Bridging Current State and New Outlooks
Edited by Patricia Bozzetto Ambrosi
p. cm.
Print ISBN 978-1-83769-958-2
Online ISBN 978-1-83769-951-3
eBook (PDF) ISBN 978-1-83769-959-9

If disposing of this product, please recycle the paper responsibly.

Meet the editor

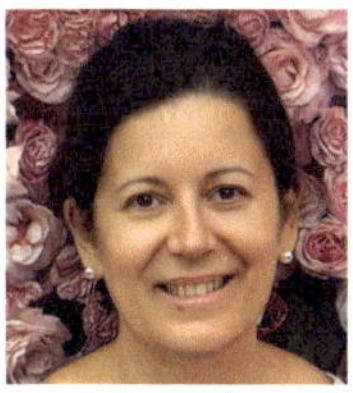

Prof. Dr. Patricia Bozzetto Ambrosi graduated in Medicine and Surgery from the University of Caxias do Sul, Brazil, and the University of Rome Tor Vergata, Italy. She is a former researcher in Morphophysiology at the University of Córdoba/Reina Sofia Hospital, Córdoba, Spain. She obtained degrees in Neurology/Neurosurgery at the Hospital of Restauração, SES, Brazil, and Neuroradiology/Radiodiagnostics at Paris Marie Curie University (Sorbonne University), France. She holds a Master's Degree in Medicine from the University of Nova Lisboa, Portugal, and a Master's Degree in Behavioral Sciences and Neuropsychiatry from the University of Pernambuco, Brazil. She also has a Ph.D. in Biological Sciences from the University of Pernambuco and Paris Diderot University. She is a former fellow in Interventional Neuroradiology at the Ophthalmological Foundation Adolphe de Rothschild, Beaujon Hospital, and Hospices Civils de Strasbourg, France. She was Praticien Associé in Interventional Neuroradiology at Neurologique Hospital Pierre Wertheimer, University of Lyon Claude Bernard, France, and a visiting professor at the University of Paris Diderot-Neuri Beaujon, France. She is an independent consultant in neuroradiology, endovascular neurology, and imaging and a Clinical Professor of Medicine. She has also been an Academic Collaborator Researcher in the Cardiovascular Department at the University of Leicester, England, and a Research Tutor at Sorbonne University, France. She has experience in innovative research for developing new technologies and neurosciences and is an academic editor and reviewer of several scientific publications about neurological diseases.

Contents

Preface

This book bridges the gap between current practices and emerging perspectives in neurological care for older adults. It serves as a valuable resource, offering both theoretical and practical frameworks for managing neurological disorders in this population while supporting their integration into clinical practice, education, and research. With the aging population growing, the prevalence of acute and chronic neurological conditions is rising. Moreover, many neurological disorders in older adults have roots in midlife or earlier, highlighting the importance of early preventive interventions.

Seven well-designed chapters of the book are divided into three sections, each reflecting an important aspect of neurological care for older adults. After the preface (available only in the printed version), the first section contains an introductory chapter describing neurological changes in the lifespan and older adults and key points in the care of older adults, such as attention to comorbidities, polypharmacy, issues involving cognitive decline, and general related support. The second section describes aspects of basic science in the clinical context in two different chapters: the first "Advanced Insights of Oxidative Stress in Ischemic Stroke: Pathogenesis, Diagnosis and Treatment" and the second "Theoretical Aspects of Protein Aggregation and Neurodegenerative Diseases". Finally, the third and most complete section contains four chapters on the most prevalent diseases affecting the elderly, related therapies, and care pathways. The fourth chapter deals with neuromuscular junction disorders in the elderly, which are divided into two major groups: primary autoimmune disease and paraneoplastic for well-defined syndromes, including Lambert Eaton myasthenic syndrome and myasthenia gravis. Primary immunologic disease has a bifid incidence peak, with both diseases found in younger individuals with a predilection for women and in older individuals with less or no gender specificity and specific challenges for older patients with myasthenic syndromes. The fifth chapter deals with vertigo, which, in addition to being a common symptom, can be caused by diseases of the peripheral and central vestibular systems that provide balance and diseases of the metabolic and vascular systems that affect the elderly population. The sixth chapter deals with emerging challenges and updates on the care pathways and pathways of chronic pain in the elderly. A comprehensive review of the concepts of pain and its consequences, as well as the most recent evidence on biological and neurological pathways of chronic pain, then focusing on the care pathways in older adults, especially in its assessment and diagnosis, multimodal interventions and interdisciplinary care that link ageing and pain, in addition to its challenges and barriers to the care pathway in older adults is also presented. In addition, ongoing research and innovations that are crucial to the advancement of chronic pain treatment in older adults will be discussed, offering new hopes for more effective and safe treatments to improve the quality of life of older adults living with chronic pain. Finally, the seventh chapter is on the role of exercise therapy in treating Parkinson's disease. This chapter describes the beneficial role of exercise therapy in treating Parkinson's disease through recent clinical empirical evidence. In addition, the chapter will describe the general exercise plan for rehabilitating patients with Parkinson's disease and an example of contemporary exercises prescribed for patients with Parkinson's disease. Finally, a brief description of the prospective research efforts needed to understand the effects of exercise therapy in reversing the pathophysiology of Parkinson's disease will be provided.

Further knowledge about neurological care in older adults is crucial both in the clinical setting and in many acute hospital admissions and long-term clinical follow-ups. Although clinicians perform the management, it is important to highlight the updated literature in this context. An opportunity to share knowledge about the latest developments in research and clinical practice. Presenting these new perspectives will lead to greater confidence in assessing and treating complex older adult patients with neurological conditions. It can also serve as a guide for integrating the knowledge base of neurological care for older adults and related skills into the education of medical students, residents, other fellows, and other medical and allied health professionals seeking regular and continuing education in this area.

Dr. Patricia Bozzetto Ambrosi
Professor,
Independent Clinical Neurology and Imaging,
Consultant,
London, United Kingdom

Clinical Professor,
European Academy of Neurology,
London, United Kingdom

American Society of Neuroradiology,
Education Committee,
London, United Kingdom

Section 1

Introduction

Chapter 1

Introductory Chapter: Neurological Disorders Burden in the Elderly and Latest Evidence in Research and Clinical Practice

Patricia Bozzetto Ambrosi

1. Introduction

Neurological disorders in older adults have become increasingly common with the world population's increasing age, resulting in many acute hospital admissions and substantial long-term disabilities, presenting challenges for healthcare systems [1, 2]. Although health professionals have become more concerned about the subject, it remains important to share updated knowledge, including these disorders' clinical features, diagnosis, and management, and highlight the literature on this context that can also assist in strategies for the prevention, treatment, and rehabilitation of these issues in the elderly [3, 4].

Aging is associated with a range of neurological changes, some of which can lead to significant health issues. These significantly impact the quality of life and pose substantial challenges in diagnosis and management [5, 6]. Common neurological conditions in the elderly include neurodegenerative diseases, cerebrovascular disorders, movement disorders, and cognitive impairments, among others listed in **Table 1**. It is important to know the most prevalent neurological disorders affecting the elderly, focusing on their clinical features, diagnosis, management, and prevention strategies to improve healthcare and the elderly population's well-being [6, 7].

2. Neurological changes burden in life span and elderly

Changes affecting the nervous system are diverse and include vascular diseases, late-onset neurodegeneration, and newly emerging conditions such as cognitive impairment following COVID-19 [3, 7]. The 2021 Global Burden of Disease study reflects global demographic and aging trends and increased exposure to environmental, metabolic, and lifestyle risk factors that are particularly relevant to noncommunicable neurological conditions such as stroke and dementia [3, 8, 9].

From one side the increased life expectancy is arguably one of the greatest achievements of health systems around the world. However, this increase has also led to increases in age-related neurological disorders, such as Alzheimer's disease and other dementias, stroke, and Parkinson's disease, necessitating global health policies not only to focus on survival but also to minimize health loss due

IntechOpen

1. Dementia
    - Alzheimer's disease (AD)
    - Vascular dementia
    - Lewy body dementia
    - Frontotemporal dementia
2. Parkinson's disease
3. Stroke
4. Neuropathies
    - Diabetic neuropathy
    - Idiopathic polyneuropathy
5. Epilepsy
6. Sleep disorders
7. *Delirium*
8. Multiple sclerosis
9. Movement disorders
    - Essential tremor
    - Restless legs syndrome
10. Neuromuscular junction disorders
    - Myasthenia gravis
    - Lambert-Eaton myasthenic syndrome
11. Common neuroinfections in the elderly
    - Bacterial meningitis
    - Viral encephalitis
    - Tuberculous meningitis
    - Fungal infections
    - Brain abscess
    - Prion diseases
    - Neurosyphilis
    - Lyme neuroborreliosis
12. Chronic pain in the elderly
    - Nociceptive pain
    - Neuropathic pain
    - Mixed pain
13. COVID related and others

Table 1.
Common neurological disorders in the elderly.

to disability by promoting function and independence. Also not all neurological burden is associated with population aging, rendering it important to quantify the overall health loss associated with nervous system conditions throughout the lifespan which is important to differentiate [10].

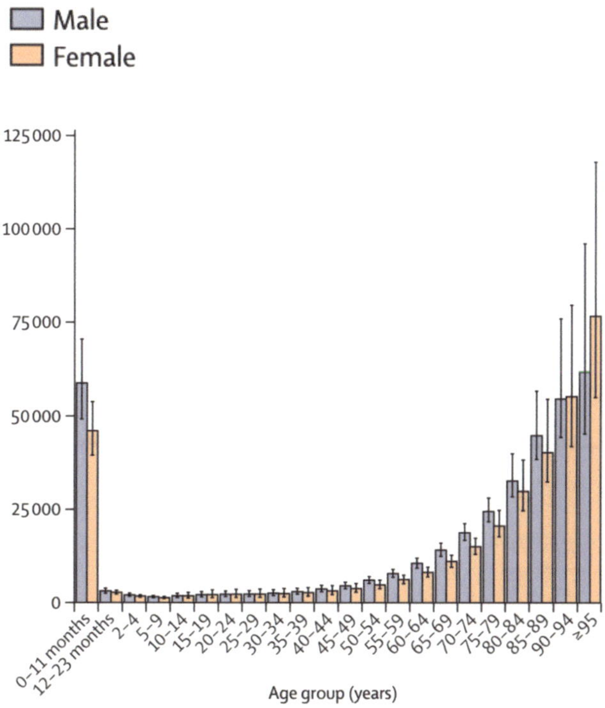

Figure 1.
Extracted from Global Study 2021 [3].

On this point, according to the 2021 Global Burden of Neurological Disease study the graph of age-standardized mortality rates, the scores of disability-adjusted life years (DALYs), and years lived with disability (YLLs) from total neurological conditions showed that it has declined [3, 7]. Also the improved public awareness of stroke and the use of statins and blood pressure-lowering medications have been linked to contributed to this decline in stroke-associated DALYs, as have, particularly in high-income countries, the approval of intravenous thrombolytics in the mid-1990s, the increasing availability of endovascular thrombectomy for acute stroke, and the growth of comprehensive stroke units [3, 7, 11, 12].

The observed reductions in DALYs were also likely driven by global vaccination and disease prevention efforts, particularly for tetanus, rabies, meningitis, neurocysticercosis and encephalitis, and improved access to prevention and treatment. However, distinct age patterns emerged for different conditions, including differences in the relative contribution of YLLs and years of healthy life lost due to disability (YLDs) to the total burden, highlighting the need for tailored interventions and prevention strategies throughout life and into old age (**Figure 1**).

Also it was observed In 2021 Global Studies that, rates of age-standardized DALYs for the total neurological category were lower in females per 100,000 people) than in males per 100,000 people; Age-specific rates show similar or higher DALY burden in males than in females in most of age groups except after 94 years old. Another important point is that neurological burden increased with age increasing.

3. Key challenges and final remarks

To finalize it will be summarizing important points in diagnosis and management of neurological changes in elderly besides the awareness to help in of these disorders:

- *Comorbidities*: Elderly patients often have multiple chronic conditions, complicating diagnosis and treatment.

- *Polypharmacy*: The use of multiple medications increases the risk of drug interactions and adverse effects.

- *Cognitive decline*: Dementia and other cognitive disorders may affect the ability to manage treatment regimens.

- *Frailty and mobility issues*: Reduced physical resilience and mobility can exacerbate neurological symptoms and impair recovery.

- *Social and Supportive needs*: The elderly may require additional social support and access to specialized care services to manage their conditions effectively.

Therefore, neurological changes in the elderly are a reality according to the major studies in literature and are multifaceted and require a comprehensive, individualized approach to diagnosis, management and life span prevention. **Early recognition, appropriate intervention, and a multidisciplinary approach** are essential to improving outcomes and quality of life for elderly patients with neurological disorders. This chapter quickly makes you aware about the common neurological problems in the elderly and familiarizes you with their unique challenges faced with their management in older adults. Then it is very important that bringing together these new perspectives will lead to increased confidence in the assessment and treatment of older patients with neurological conditions.

Acknowledgements

I acknowledge the use of ChatGPT-3.5 (Open AI, Available from: https://chat.openai.com/) to summarize the common neurological disorders listed on **Table 1** and key challenges listed on Final Remarks.

Conflict of interest

P.B.A. declared no conflict of interest to disclose.

Acronyms and abbreviations

AD	Alzheimer's disease
DALYs	disability-adjusted life years
YLLs	years lived with disability

Author details

Patricia Bozzetto Ambrosi
Neurology and Clinical Medicine, Fellow of the European Academy of Neurology, Radiology and Neuroimaging at Sorbonne University, France

*Address all correspondence to: patricia.ambrosi@icloud.com

References

[1] Hou Y, Dan X, Babbar M, Wei Y, Hasselbalch SG, Croteau DL, et al. Ageing as a risk factor for neurodegenerative disease. Nature Reviews Neurology. 2019;**15**(10):565-581

[2] Stanton BR. The neurology of old age. Clinical Medicine. 2011;**11**(1):54-56

[3] Articles Global, Regional, and National Burden of Disorders Affecting the Nervous System, 1990-2021: A Systematic Analysis for the Global Burden of Disease Study 2021 GBD 2021 Nervous System Disorders Collaborators

[4] Bernhardt J, Duncan PW, Lynch E. Improving access to, and quality of stroke rehabilitation. Stroke. 2023;**54**(9):2446-2448

[5] Steinmetz JD, Seeher KM, Schiess N, Nichols E, Cao B, Servili C, et al. Global, regional, and national burden of disorders affecting the nervous system, 1990-2021: A systematic analysis for the global burden of disease study 2021. The Lancet Neurology. 2024;**23**(4):344-381

[6] Nur D, Kung W. Challenges and perspectives of neurological disorders. Brain Sciences. 2023;**13**(4):676-676

[7] Intersectoral Global Action Plan on Epilepsy and Other Neurological Disorders [Internet]. www.who.int. Available from: https://www.who.int/publications/i/item/9789240076624

[8] Feigin VL, Stark BA, Johnson CO, Roth GA, Bisignano C, Abady GG, et al. Global, regional, and national burden of stroke and its risk factors, 1990-2019: A systematic analysis for the global burden of disease study 2019. The Lancet Neurology. 2021;**20**(10):795-820. Available from: https://www.thelancet.com/journals/laneur/article/PIIS1474-4422(21)00252-0/fulltext

[9] GBD. 2019 dementia forecasting collaborators. Estimation of the global prevalence of dementia in 2019 and forecasted prevalence in 2050: An analysis for the global burden of disease study 2019. The Lancet Public Health. 2022;**7**(2):e105-e125. DOI: 10.1016/S2468-2667(21)00249-8

[10] Feigin VL, Nichols E, Alam T, Bannick MS, Beghi E, Blake N, et al. Global, regional, and national burden of neurological disorders, 1990-2016: A systematic analysis for the global burden of disease study 2016. The Lancet Neurology. 2019;**18**(5):459-480. Available from: https://www.sciencedirect.com/science/article/pii/S147444221830499X

[11] Amarenco P, Labreuche J. Lipid management in the prevention of stroke: Review and updated meta-analysis of statins for stroke prevention. The Lancet Neurology. 2009;**8**(5):453-463. Available from: https://www.ncbi.nlm.nih.gov/pubmed/19375663

[12] Goyal M, Demchuk AM, Menon BK, Eesa M, Rempel JL, Thornton J, et al. Randomized assessment of rapid endovascular treatment of ischemic stroke. New England Journal of Medicine. 2015;**372**(11):1019-1030

Section 2

Basic Science in Clinical Context

Chapter 2

Advanced Insights of Oxidative Stress in Ischemic Stroke: Pathogenesis, Diagnosis and Treatment

Qiyi Yu, Yidong Zhang, Yifan Wu, Xianda Ma and Yuxiao Chen

Abstract

Ischemic stroke is one of the major causes of disability and mortality in the aged people. A better understanding of the pathology, mechanism, diagnosis and treatment of stroke might have important practical implications for patient clinical management, especially for aged patients. Affected by cerebral ischemia, neurons are not capable of maintaining cellular respiration metabolism, leading to excitotoxicity and calcium overload, which further induce oxidative stress. During oxidative stress process, the reactive oxygen species is massively produced, which involved in the regulation of diverse biological processes including lipid, DNA, protein and signaling pathways. This review is aimed to provide a comprehensive overview of oxidative stress in ischemic stroke, particularly ischemic stroke occurred in the elderly. Our topics included the pathogenesis and the role oxidative stress plays in the ischemic stroke occurrence and development. Additionally, oxidative stress-related diagnostic methods and antioxidant therapies in clinical use are further discussed. With a focus perspective on aged patients, we expect our review can contribute to guide a comprehensive acknowledgment of oxidative stress in ischemic stroke, suggesting preventive treatment toward antioxidant-based therapy as a novel therapeutic alternative for the elderly.

Keywords: oxidative stress, ischemic stroke, neuron death, stroke diagnosis, antioxidant therapies

1. Introduction

Stroke is one of the main reasons for disability and mortality in aged people, accounting for over 12 million new cases and 6 million deaths globally per year [1]. Defined as a syndrome of acute and focal neurological deficit caused by vascular injury to the central nervous system, stroke is mainly divided into two types: hemorrhagic stroke (HS) and ischemic stroke (IS) [2]. HS is triggered by damage to brain blood vessels, while IS the consequence of the blockage of brain arteries. Although both forms are prevalent worldwide, IS represents 70–80% of all stroke cases [3–5]. Approximately 80% of strokes occur in individuals aged 65 years and older, with the occurrence of stroke doubling each decade after the age of 55 [6]. Older patients not only exhibit a higher incidence of stroke but also experience increased mortality rates, more severe neurological deficits and slower recovery compared to younger individuals [7].

Mechanistically, caused by the blockage of brain blood vessels, cerebral ischemia is a condition indicating restricted blood supplement in the brain, which results in reduced oxygen and nutrients for brain tissue [8, 9]. Affected by cerebral ischemia, neurons are not capable of maintaining cellular oxidative metabolism, disrupting normal cell metabolism and oxidative stress, even causing cell death [10]. Brain tissue is especially prone to oxidative stress resulting from several factors [11]. Neurons contain high concentrations of polyunsaturated fatty acids, which can be easily peroxidized by free radicals, thereby triggering oxidative stress, given the low proportion of antioxidant enzymes [12, 13]. It is reported that ischemia stimulates the generation of nitric oxide (NO) from the vascular endothelial cells to increase local blood flow [14, 15]. However, the excessive release of NO could bring negative outcomes, like release of free oxygen radicals and peroxynitrite anion ($ONOO^-$). $ONOO^-$ is characterized as an effective oxidizing agent that promotes DNA damage and lipid peroxidation in neurons. Thus, oxidative stress is a significant component in IS pathogenesis [16, 17].

2. Pathogenesis of ischemic stroke

2.1 Thrombosis and blood flow occlusion

Aging exerts a significant impact on the brain microvasculature. Alterations in the composition of connective tissues and muscles of vessel walls are observed with aging, leading to cerebral hypoperfusion and thrombosis [18, 19]. Meanwhile, the structural modifications in choroid plexuses are also evidenced. These changes jointly include thickening of the basement membrane, fibrosis and amyloidal deposition in the choroid blood vessels, resulting in a decrease of cerebrospinal fluid secretion and turnover [20]. Aging typically leads to large vessel atherosclerosis, vasculitis and arterial dissection, which are also common risk factors that contribute to thrombosis [21–23].

Cerebral thrombosis blocks blood supplements to neurons, and the decreased cerebral blood flow (CBF) also triggers blood vessel dilation for autoregulation through the release of vasoactive substances, such as NO. However, the senescent brain endothelial cells promote neurovascular uncoupling by deregulating angiogenesis and vascular endothelial growth factor (VEGF) or by increasing ROS and reducing NO production [24]. The changed brain microvasculature further worsens the dysregulation of CBF, particularly under ischemic conditions.

When the excessive decline in perfusion pressure of CBF exceeds the brain's ability of compensation, CBF continues to diminish and various biological processes become dysregulated [25]. Protein synthesis starts to cease if the CBF rate is ≤50 ml/100 g/min and ceases thoroughly at 35 ml/100 g/min with transient increase in glucose metabolism. The glucose utilization declines sharply when CBF decreases to 25 ml/100 g/min, and the glycolysis process ensues [26]. Glycolysis produces lactic acid, which leads to tissue acidosis if lactic acid accumulates. As CBF continues to drop to 16–18 ml/100 g/min, the neuronal electrical failure occurs, then the loss of membrane ion homeostasis at 10–12 ml/100 g/min, which typically indicates the occurrence of infarction.

2.2 Excitotoxicity and calcium overload

In IS, the blood flow is interrupted after the occurrence of thrombosis, which causes a decline in oxygen and nutrient supply [27]. With low levels of oxygen and metabolic substrates, aerobic respiration is inhibited, resulting in severe adenosine triphosphate (ATP) deficiency in brain tissue [28]. Lacking ATP, the ATP-dependent ion channels located in the membrane, especially Na^+/K^+ ATPase, become dysregulated and cannot maintain the membrane electrochemical gradient, causing continuous depolarization of glia and neurons [28, 29]. Meanwhile, the dysregulated Ca^{2+} pump, along with ATP deficiency, switches the voltage-controlled Ca^{2+} ion channels, eventually stimulating the increase in Ca^{2+} concentration in neurons.

Increased Ca^{2+} levels in cells triggers the secretion of excitatory neurotransmitters, especially glutamate. Due to ATP deficiency, the reuptake of extracellular glutamate is suppressed, causing excessive glutamate to accumulate in extracellular space. The free glutamate binds to the ionotropic receptors, especially N-methyl-d-aspartic acid (NMDA) and α-amino-3-hydroxy-5-methyl-4-isoxazolepropionic acid (AMPA) present at the postsynaptic neurons, causing extensive Ca^{2+} influx and subsequent calcium overload. The sustained Ca^{2+} influx activates the phospholipases and proteases in neurons. The generation of the ROS is also stimulated. Activation of phospholipases promotes the disintegration of biological membranes, allowing H_2O to enter into the cell. Additionally, glutamate-mediated overstimulation allows the influx of Na^+ and Cl^- into the cell [30]. The inward movement of water molecules and Na^+ induces cell swelling, cytotoxic edema and necrosis, resulting in neuron damage.

Besides, the sustained Ca^{2+} influx promotes the dysregulation of mitochondria [31, 32]. The dysregulation of mitochondria in neurons stimulates alternation of membrane permeability, mitochondria swelling and collapse, consequently, the activation of apoptotic as well as oxidative stress pathways [33]. Apart from glutamate receptors, there are also other ion channels involved in calcium overload during ischemia, like Na^+/Ca^{2+} exchanger and acid-sensing ion channels [34, 35]. Aging exacerbates mitochondrial fusion, leading to progressive alterations in mitochondrial dynamics and function, presumably to buffer increased Ca^{2+} load and ROS production [36]. However, these adaptive adjustments become detrimental under ischemic conditions, leading to increased and early glutamate release and a rapid exhaustion of mitochondrial capacity to sustain energy status of axons.

3. Oxidative stress in ischemic stroke

During aerobic respiration, ATP is primarily generated in the mitochondria through oxidative phosphorylation, a process that also produces a small but continuous amount of ROS, specifically superoxide (O_2^-), within the mitochondrial matrix [37, 38]. In elderly populations, the efficiency of mitochondrial oxidative phosphorylation declines, leading to increased baseline ROS production and heightened vulnerability to oxidative damage [39]. Under normal physiological conditions, this superoxide is rapidly converted to hydrogen peroxide (H_2O_2) by the enzyme superoxide dismutase (SOD), allowing H_2O_2 to act as an intracellular messenger in cellular signaling pathways [40]. However, during IS, the oxygen supply is rapidly depleted before glucose, forcing cells to rely on glycolysis for ATP production in the absence of sufficient oxygen. This shift to anaerobic metabolism leads to the accumulation of lactic acid, a byproduct of glycolysis, within brain tissue [41]. The excessive lactic acid accumulation not only disrupts cellular pH balance, contributing to acidosis but also promotes a pro-oxidant environment in neurons, which intensifies oxidative stress [42].

Furthermore, in ischemic conditions, the antioxidant defenses in neurons, including enzymes such as SOD, glutathione peroxidase and catalase, become inactivated or overwhelmed due to ROS overproduction and the depletion of cellular antioxidants. Age-related reductions in antioxidant enzyme activity further impair the ability of elderly neurons to neutralize ROS, accelerating oxidative damage. This impairment of the antioxidant system, combined with the release of oxidative ions from cellular proteins, exacerbates ROS accumulation, leading to significant cellular and mitochondrial damage [43]. In the ischemic environment, neurons are particularly vulnerable to oxidative stress for their high metabolic rate and the high content of polyunsaturated fatty acids in their membranes, which are susceptible to peroxidation by ROS. Additionally, the high content of polyunsaturated fatty acids in elderly neuronal membranes is especially prone to peroxidation, amplifying membrane destabilization during stroke [12, 13]. The cumulative effect of dysregulated mitochondrial process and inactivated antioxidant defenses contributes to the progressive damage seen in IS, including cellular swelling, membrane destabilization and, ultimately, cell death.

Apart from the dysregulated mitochondrial activity, another significant contributor to reactive oxygen species is the enzyme nicotinamide adenine dinucleotide phosphate (NADPH) oxidase (NOX), which plays a crucial role in the development of oxidative stress and subsequent injury, particularly in IS and cerebral ischemia-reperfusion injury [44]. NOX generates ROS by transferring electrons from NADPH to oxygen molecules, producing superoxide, which can further convert into H_2O_2 and other reactive species, thereby intensifying oxidative stress. Following cerebral ischemia, NOX activity significantly increases, with one of the NOX isoforms, NOX4, showing particularly marked upregulation within hours. Research indicates that NOX4 expression in neurons and vascular structures peaks approximately 24 hours post-ischemic injury [45, 46]. In the reperfusion phase, the sustained elevation of NOX4 expression leads to excessive ROS production, which exacerbates neuronal damage. Furthermore, ROS generated by NOX can activate various proinflammatory molecules and signaling pathways, such as the nuclear factor kappa B (NF-κB) pathway, triggering neuron inflammatory reactions [47]. This process recruits proinflammatory cells, including neutrophils and macrophages, to the affected area, which releases additional ROS and proinflammatory factors, amplifying oxidative stress and neuroinflammation.

3.1 Biological effects of excessive ROS in IS

ROS have various biological effects, such as stimulating neuron injury and death, including lipid peroxidation, protein denaturation, DNA modification and disruption of signaling pathways [48]. Many of them have detrimental effects of accumulated ROS exceeding the compensatory ability of antioxidant defenses.

3.1.1 Lipid peroxidation

Lipid peroxidation, initiated by ROS attacking polyunsaturated fatty acids in cell membranes, plays a critical role in cellular injury. Lipid peroxides generated in this process are highly reactive, further intensifying cellular damage by compromising membrane integrity and fluidity, increasing permeability and disrupting essential cellular functions [49]. Lipid peroxidation in IS induces the generation of conjugated dienic hydroperoxides that are further decomposed into aldehydes, dienals, or alkanes. For example, the membrane phospholipids are hydrolyzed by phospholipase A2, and the fatty acids are released freely, like arachidonic acid (AA) [50]. ROS is produced in AA metabolism process, which reacts with lipids to form lipid peroxidation products [51]. In stroke, increased levels of phospholipase A2 have been observed in serum, indicating the upregulation of AA metabolism and ROS production. Additionally, the downstream metabolic products, 4-hydroxynonenal (HNE) damages neurons and white matter, eventually triggering apoptotic pathways [52]. The immunoreactive response of HNE in the ipsilateral striatum shows a significant correlation with focal ischemia in rats [53]. These reactive aldehydes can form covalent adducts with cellular proteins and nucleic acids, leading to cellular dysfunction and amplifying oxidative stress by promoting a cycle of free radical formation and continuous lipid damage [54].

3.1.2 Protein denaturation

High levels of ROS result in oxidative modifications to proteins, including denaturation and degradation, which can severely compromise protein function and structural integrity [55]. These oxidative changes often lead to protein misfolding and aggregation, rendering enzymes, receptors and structural proteins particularly vulnerable [56]. The disruption of these proteins impairs vital cellular processes, such as metabolism, signal transduction and cellular architecture maintenance. Moreover, oxidized proteins tend to form insoluble aggregates within neurons, which not only contribute to cellular stress but may also accelerate neurodegenerative processes [55, 57].

3.1.3 DNA modifications

ROS-induced DNA damage encompasses strand breaks, base modifications and cross-linking, which trigger a series of detrimental effects within cells. Oxidative lesions in both nuclear and mitochondrial DNA activate repair enzymes that consume substantial cellular energy, thereby exacerbating ATP consumption [58]. Persistent DNA damage leads to mutations, impaired gene expression and the activation of cell death pathways. In neurons, which highly rely on stable gene expression for their function, ROS-induced DNA damage is particularly harmful, contributing to long-term dysfunction and cell death [58]. In IS, nuclear DNA damage occurs through two main mechanisms: oxidative stress modifications and endonuclease-mediated DNA fragmentation [59]. DNA oxidation activates repair enzymes, such as poly (ADP-ribose) polymerase (PARP), which, while repairing damage, consume large amounts of cellular energy and exacerbate neuronal ATP depletion. This worsens oxygen and energy imbalances within neurons, intensifying cellular stress. Currently, a decrease in the nucleoprotein apurinic/apyrimidinic endonuclease (APE/Ref-1) has been shown to inhibit DNA oxidation processes. APE/Ref-1, an essential component of the DNA base repair pathway, regulates various transcription factors by cleaving ROS-induced apyrimidinic sites, thus playing a protective role against oxidative DNA damage [60, 61].

3.1.4 Cell signaling effects of ROS

Via redox-sensitive signaling pathways, the ROS poses diverse effects on cellular processes. ROS generated in mitochondria induces the release of cytochrome c, which further combines with apoptotic protease activating factor 1 (Apaf-1) and deoxyadenosine triphosphate, contributing to the formation of apoptosome [62]. Meanwhile, caspase-9 is activated, followed by the activation of caspase-3. Caspase-3 is an enzyme that cleaves nuclear DNA repair enzymes [63]. The activation of caspase-3 leads to a boost in oxidative DNA lesions in neuron cells [64]. In cortical lesion mouse models, antioxidant therapy was evidenced to inhibit caspase-3 intensity, thus inhibiting DNA fragmentation and brain lesion development [63].

Ischemia in cerebral regions has been shown to induce the phosphorylation and translocation of the B-cell lymphoma 2 (BCL-2) to mitochondria, a process where ROS plays a pivotal role [65]. Additionally, the p53-regulated modulator of apoptosis (PUMA) contributes to the apoptotic cascade by interacting with BCL-2, making it another potential mediator of neuronal death in IS [66]. *In vivo* studies reveal that PUMA expression is upregulated in hippocampal neurons following transient ischemia, indicating its contributing role in IS development [67]. However, the apoptosis effect triggered by ROS can be mitigated through phosphorylation by the phosphatidylinositol-3-kinase (PI3K)/Akt pathway [68]. Experimental data from cerebral rat synaptosomes exposed to oxidants indicate that the PI3K/Akt pathway is significantly upregulated, evidenced by an acute and transient increase in phosphoinositide-kinase (PPI) labeling. Moreover, treatment with LY294002, a PI3K/Akt pathway inhibitor, was shown to prevent the oxidative activation of PPI and PI3K, resulting in the upregulation of phosphorylation level of BCL-2. The results suggested that PI3K/Akt pathway modulation may provide a protective effect against ROS-induced apoptosis in ischemic conditions [69].

NF-κB represents another crucial signaling pathway in IS that is activated in response to oxidative stress, inflammation and cellular damage [70]. When oxidative stress occurs, the generation of ROS will trigger the activation of NF-κB pathway, causing neuronal cell death and triggering inflammatory pathways, eventually worsening the process of neurodegeneration and cellular damage. Xyloketal B inhibited the ROS/TLR4/NF-κB pathway, resulting in reduced cerebral infarction in MCAO mice. In mice with IS, Bergenin exhibited neuroprotective effects by inhibiting oxidative stress by regulating SIRT1/Forkhead box protein O3a/NF-κB pathway [71]. To sum up, the occurrence of oxidative stress is strongly linked to the activation of NF-κB in IS.

Furthermore, ischemic conditions have been shown to activate the erk1/2 pathway in primary mouse endothelial cells, a process facilitated by VEGF induction [72]. This upregulation is thought to promote cell survival and angiogenesis, highlighting the interplay between ischemic signaling and repair mechanisms. In addition to NF-κB, other transcription factors and signaling pathways—such as p38, JNK and heat shock factor 1—are also activated in response to ROS and contribute to the complex network of cellular responses in IS [73]. These pathways collectively influence inflammation, apoptosis and cellular repair, underscoring the multifaceted role of ROS-sensitive signaling in IS pathology.

3.2 Nitric oxide synthases (NOS) and NO in ischemic stroke

NO is synthesized *via* biological processes catalyzed by nitric oxide synthases (NOS). The NOS expressed in the central nervous system can be characterized as three types: neuronal NOS (nNOS), endothelial NOS (eNOS) and inducible NOS (iNOS) [74]. nNOS and eNOS are Ca^{2+} dependent, and iNOS is Ca^{2+} independent [75].

During the early stage of IS, decreased CBF first triggers the activation of eNOS, promoting NO release for regulation of CBF and protection of brain micro-vessels. In eNOS-related genes knock-out mice, the infarct size was larger compared with wild-type mice [76]. However, the continued CBF decrease induces excitotoxicity and Ca^{2+} overload, which mainly regulates the Ca^{2+}-dependent NOS, nNOS, to release excessive NO, exerting neurotoxic effects. iNOS is activated from 12 hours after IS occurrence, and it is mainly generated by microglia, astrocytes, endothelial cells and infiltrating lymphocytes [77]. The NO release caused by iNOS is around 1000 times that of NO by nNOS, exhibiting a stronger neurotoxic effect [78]. Additionally, the production of NO induced by iNOS also leads to further brain damage during reperfusion after ischemia [79]. The ischemia mouse models that received knockdown of nNOS-related or iNOS-related genes exhibited general neuroprotective effects [80, 81].

In addition, NO might also participate in the breakdown of blood-brain barrier (BBB) after IS. The components of BBB are the astrocytic end-feet, extracellular matrix and endothelials. These components are linked tightly by the junction adhesion molecule-1 (JAM1), claudins and occludins [82]. The cytoplasmic domains of these cells are attached to the cytoskeleton *via* attached proteins [74]. However, the barrier structure is weakened by matrix metalloproteinases (MMPs) *via* hydrolysis of the junction and extracellular matrix proteins, with the rapid increase of MMP-2 expression after brain ischemia, followed by the MMP-9 activation [83, 84]. Despite the unclearness of exact molecular mechanism, mounting evidence has confirmed that internal NO release facilitates the BBB disruption induced by brain [16]. Previous research demonstrated that endogenous NO produced by NOS contributes to BBB disruption by modulating the activity of MMPs during brain I/R, as the permeability of BBB in rats increased significantly during cerebral ischemia and reperfusion, accompanied by the upregulation of MMPs and downregulation of tight junction protein zonula occludens-1 in the rat brain, which could be reversed by L-NAME, a type of NOS inhibitor [85]. Further, through the reaction with superoxide, NO promotes the generation of $ONOO^-$, a high-intensive radical that can easily penetrate lipid membranes [86]. $ONOO^-$ exerts neurotoxic effects through lipid peroxidation, protein tyrosine nitration, PARP activation and promotion of mitochondrial dysfunction [87].

3.3 Oxidative stress in aging

The preceding sections demonstrated the close associations between oxidative stress and IS. Moreover, numerous studies have proved that aging or senescence is a risk factor that aggravates stroke. Therefore, it can be assumed that oxidative stress and stroke are more prevalent in the elderly population.

The close link between oxidative stress and aging can be evidenced by several relevant mechanisms [88, 89]. For example, the increased oxidative stress and neuroinflammation activity in aging hippocampus induce cognitive decline, reduced neurogenesis and synaptic plasticity [90]. Moreover, the mutual impacts of neuroinflammation and oxidative stress further exacerbate the aging process [91]. Here, neuroinflammation stimulates both macrophage and microglia, which produce extra ROS in the mitochondrial matrix, increasing the burden of antioxidant defenses in neurons.

As previously described, aging involves a series of pathological events related to declined physiological functions, including thinner brain microvasculature, DNA damage, shortened telomeres and reduced immune responses [92]. When exposed to ischemia, aging impairs the integrity of the neurovascular unit and damages brain tissues [93]. Aging can also destroy collateral circulation and revascularization of the brain through increased free radical and inflammatory responses to aggravate stroke [94]. Additionally, alterations in molecules and signaling pathways associated with aging have also been identified. E2F1 has been shown to promote cellular senescence in human fibroblasts, whereas transcription factor FOXO3 counteracts senescence by regulating ROS-scavenging proteins. E2F1 can directly bind to FOXO3 in the nucleus, inhibiting FOXO3-dependent transcription and accelerating the aging process [95, 96].

Thus, when stroke occurs, excessive generation of ROS follows, leading to cellular damage and brain injury. Subsequently, oxidative stress and the overloaded antioxidant system jointly contributed to the accumulation of ROS, followed by brain deterioration. Aging acts as a key risk factor in the stroke process, as the declined physiological brain functions can largely aggravate the development of stroke.

4. Diagnosis after IS

The immediate medical care of IS after the occurrence, and proper diagnostic methods are critical for the stabilization of patients [97–99]. To accurately and timely identify the symptoms of stroke, several medical techniques have been applied to clinical practice. For precise assessment, brain scanning and imaging are promising practices and are essential for final confirmation after blood detection. Neuroimaging assists physicians in developing proper strategies for treatment. Computed tomography (CT) has been utilized widely in clinical practice. CT scans can identify slight lesions in cytotoxic edema, alterations in gray-white matter areas, hypoattenuation of basal ganglia, tissue swelling and blood vessel occlusion [100, 101]. Apart from CT, magnetic resonance imaging (MRI) or advanced imaging techniques, such as magnetic resonance perfusion, are also widely adopted.

One dilemma of stroke diagnosis and treatment is wake-up stroke. Wake-up stroke usually occurs in sleep and accounts for a proportion of 25% of stroke cases [102, 103]. Although rtPA therapy is widely used in stroke management, the therapeutic window might have been surpassed. Also, CT or MRI techniques are not immediately available. In this situation, the diagnostic indexes that are simple, accessible and highly specific can help to identify patients with IS rapidly and screen those who are suitable or not suitable for reperfusion therapy [104].

Clinically, a single onset of stroke carries the risk of permanent disability, and the thrombus formed in brain vessels and reocclusion in arterials indicate fatal recurrence [105, 106]. Thus, reduction of stroke-associated mortality is crucial [13, 107]. In general, some laboratory biomarkers have been adopted for the evaluation of prognosis of acute IS or reperfusion [108]. Since ROS production is strongly associated with the mechanism of stroke, the relevant redox biomarkers are potent indexes for evaluation of IS development and prognosis of IS patients [109, 110]. Notably, the redox reactions participate in various diseases and the corresponding biomarkers might vary; it is imprecise to monitor and evaluate the IS development according to only one single biomarker.

So far, researchers have successfully established specific redox biomarkers that are significantly correlated with stroke incidence [111]. In elderly patients, oxidative stress biomarkers tend to exhibit more pronounced variations, reflecting the exacerbated oxidative damage associated with aging and comorbidities. Variations in levels of lipids, DNA, enzymes and protein oxidation are identified as potential biomarkers for IS [112]. Studies indicate that the severity of oxidative stress could influence prognosis and clinical outcomes of an acute IS patient, especially in dimensions of cognition and mortality risk. For example, it has been demonstrated that a linear regression model could describe the relationship between oxidized low-density lipoprotein levels in plasma and post-stroke cognition of patients, which was assessed by the scores of mental state examination [110]. Moreover, their findings revealed that a higher risk of death or poor cognition was correlated with elevated oxidized low-density lipoprotein levels in stroke patients, especially when associated with large-artery atherosclerosis [113]. This relationship is particularly relevant for the elderly population, where large-artery atherosclerosis is more prevalent and significantly contributes to poorer outcomes. *Via* bioinformatic analysis of bulk-seq mRNA expression profiles of IS patients, the biomarker genes have been identified from peripheral blood, with a receiver operating characteristic curve of 0.940 [114]. In elderly individuals, the identification of these biomarkers could help tailor personalized therapeutic strategies, accounting for age-specific oxidative stress dynamics. Biomarkers in peripheral blood is widely applied for evaluation of diagnosis and treatment in clinical usage, which is rapid and easy to access compared with other samples. The peripheral blood biomarkers associate the oxidative stress development in IS with peripheral variations, which is promising to new IS diagnosis methods and treatment therapies [115].

5. Clinical antioxidant treatment strategies in IS

Being a critical biological process in IS, oxidative stress exerts severe consequences, including neuron apoptosis, tissue damage and the function impairment that might be irreversible [116]. Thus, antioxidant treatments are essential. In normal physiological metabolisms in the brain, the formation and consumption of ROS are balanced by inner antioxidant mechanisms and processes. However, after the onset of stroke, free radicals are produced massively, overwhelming the body's antioxidant systems. Considering that elderly individuals are more susceptible to strokes and often have weakened antioxidant defenses due to aging, targeted therapeutic strategies are particularly important for this population. Antioxidant treatments for elderly patients should taking both the excessive production of ROS and the age-related declines in cellular repair mechanisms and mitochondrial function into consideration. Thus, enhancing the processes of ROS scavenging and degradation is crucial to restoring oxidative balance and mitigating the damage caused by oxidative stress. Here, there are three primary treatment strategies for antioxidant function through three mechanisms to address the excessive ROS: ROS production inhibition, ROS scavenging and promotion of ROS degradation [117].

5.1 Inhibition of ROS production

This approach aims to inhibit the production of ROS by specifically targeting the enzymes related to ROS generation. The two main targets that are mostly applied in the clinical treatment of stroke are NOX and xanthine oxidase (XO). NOX catalyzes production reactions of superoxide, therefore inhibiting NOX is a clinical treatment strategy for stroke. In elderly patients, the upregulation of NOX activity has been observed to be more pronounced, potentially due to age-related vascular dysfunction and chronic inflammation, making NOX inhibition particularly significant for this population. Apocynin, one non-specific antioxidant, has been evidenced to protect the brain against neuron injury after MCAO and to reduce the infarct size as well as

BCL-2 levels [118, 119]. Apocynin also suppresses the activity of Rho kinase; thus, the p47phox subunit cannot migrate to the membrane, and NOX complex cannot assemble [120, 121]. VAS2870, another inhibitor of NOX, also has been shown to inhibit infarct development, oxidative stress development, neuronal apoptosis and BBB damage [122]. However, most NOX inhibitors lack isoform selectivity, an area where more specific inhibitors could offer insights into the distinct roles of NOX isoforms in IS.

In ischemic conditions, ATP depletion also leads to the accumulation of hypoxanthine and xanthine, substrates for XO. Through proteolytic cleavage, xanthine dehydrogenase converts to XO, increasing ROS production [123]. Allopurinol, and its metabolite oxypurinol, have been utilized as inhibitors of hydroxyl radical production [124]. The infarct size was observed to reduce by around 35% after treatment with allopurinol, along with significant reductions in neurological impairment and mortality [125].

5.2 Free radical scavengers

In infarcted brains, the ischemia induces the Ca^{2+} overload and activates phospholipase A2, which enables the release of free fatty acids, especially AA [126]. ROS is produced in the process of AA metabolism, which reacts with lipids to form lipid peroxides, leading to a burst of free radicals in ischemic penumbra areas [127]. Edaravone, a derivative of 2-pyrazolin-5-one, has a similar activity to phenol. Edaravone has been observed to show a high intensity of free radical removal by quenching hydroxyl radicals ($^{\bullet}OH$) and inhibiting $^{\bullet}OH$-dependent and $^{\bullet}OH$-independent lipid peroxidation [128]. According to a multi-center clinical trial, edaravone showed protective effects in humans 3 months after IS without severe side effects, especially exhibited a significant reduction in infarct size and improved post-stroke functional recovery in the aged patients [129]. Currently, edaravone has been approved in Japan as the neuroprotective agent for IS patients.

Also, the supplementation of antioxidants can contribute to the clearance of ROS [116]. Vitamin C (ascorbate, ascorbic acid) is an effective antioxidant that can directly scavenge ROS and nitrogen-based radicals. Additionally, Vitamin C boosts the activity of eNOS and inhibits the activity of NOX. The antioxidant characteristics of Vitamin C are improved in combination treatment strategies, for example, the combined use of vitamins C and E [130]. Experiments have evidenced that higher Vitamin C concentration in serum is correlated with a lower risk of IS [131]. In summary, the higher the vitamin C level, the lower the IS risk and lipid peroxidation extent.

5.3 Free radical degradation

The degradation of free radicals represents a crucial component of antioxidant therapies, which aim to neutralize existing ROS within cells. SOD catalyzes the conversion of O_2^- into H_2O_2, which is then further degraded by catalase (CAT) and glutathione peroxidase (GSH-Px), reducing oxidative damage. Three SOD isoforms participate in this process, with SOD1 being the primary focus of clinical research [132, 133]. Studies have shown that overexpression of SOD1 in transgenic mice and rats decreases neuronal apoptosis, underscoring its potential protective role against ischemic injury. Another significant target in free radical degradation is NO, a vasoactive molecule that, when derived from iNOS, can interact with superoxide to form $ONOO^-$, which exerts neurotoxic effects through mechanisms such as lipid peroxidation, protein tyrosine nitration and activation of PARP, all of which contribute to cell damage and apoptosis [134]. Elderly patients tend to present with elevated levels of $ONOO^-$, further highlighting the importance of therapies targeting its neutralization in this population. The compound lubeluzole has shown promise as an NO modulator by downregulating NO levels, thereby reducing $ONOO^-$ accumulation. Pre-clinical studies have indicated lubeluzole's potential efficacy in mitigating neurotoxic effects associated with $ONOO^-$, though further research is required to confirm its clinical benefits [135].

5.4 Mitochondria-targeted antioxidant therapies

Mitochondrial matrix is also a typical source of free radicals in IS. The damaged mitochondria during oxidative stress can trigger upregulated ROS production and reduced ATP production, as well as the promotion of cell apoptosis. The inhibition of mitochondrial respiratory chain complex I was identified to benefit neurons in stroke treatment [136]. Due to the difficulty of maintaining high levels of antioxidants in intracellular space, therapy targeting ROS generated in mitochondria is complicated. Currently, there are solutions to address the problem. By conjugating an antioxidant with a lipophilic cation, the antioxidant diffuses and accumulates in the targeted regions [137]. Mitoquinone, a derivative of ubiquinone, has been shown to protect mitochondria from the oxidative damage caused by H_2O_2 [138].

6. Conclusion

Generally, in this review, we comprehensively discussed the key role of oxidative stress that plays after the onset of IS, including the production, function and biological effects that oxidative stress poses to neurons in IS. Positive feedback between oxidative stress and IS development usually exists after the onset of stroke, and targeting oxidative stress might offer novel diagnostic and treatment strategies to prevent stroke occurrence and development. However, given the complicated interactions between various cascades that promote the injury of neurons after cerebral ischemia and reperfusion, more studies focusing on the oxidative stress process in IS are still needed. With the development of clinical and experimental techniques, further research into oxidative stress and in-depth mechanisms is promising to bring a new perspective for IS. As research continues to advance, new therapies and management strategies hold the promise of enhancing the quality of life of IS patients, especially those elderly patients.

Acknowledgements

Thanks to all participants in this study.

Authorship contribution statement

Qiyi Yu: Conception, manuscript reviewing; Yidong Zhang: Manuscript draft; Yifan Wu: article collection, manuscript reviewing; Yuxiao Chen: Manuscript draft; Xianda Ma: Manuscript reviewing.

Conflict of interest

The authors declare that the research was conducted in the absence of any commercial or financial relationships that could be construed as a potential conflict of interest.

Abbreviations

HS	hemorrhagic stroke
IS	ischemic stroke
NO	nitric oxide
$ONOO^-$	peroxynitrite anion
CBF	cerebral blood flow
ATP	adenosine triphosphate
NMDA	N-methyl-d-aspartic acid
AMPA	α-amino-3-hydroxy-5-methyl-4-isoxazolepropionic acid
ROS	reactive oxygen species
SOD	superoxide dismutase
NAPDH	nicotinamide adenine dinucleotide phosphate
NOX	NAPDH-oxidase
MCAO	middle cerebral artery occlusion
CK2	casein kinase 2
HNE	4-hydroxynonenal
AA	arachidonic acid
PARP	poly ADP-ribose polymerase
APE/Ref-1	apurinic apyrimidinic endonuclease
Apaf-1	apoptotic protease activating factor 1
BCL-2	B-cell lymphoma 2
BAD	BCL-2 associated death promoter
PUMA	P53-regulated modulator of apoptosis
PI3K	phosphatidylinositol-3-kinase
PPI	phosphoinositide-kinase
NOS	nitric oxide synthases
nNOS	neuron NOS
eNOS	endothelial NOS
iNOS	inducible NOS
BBB	blood-brain barrier
JAM1	junction adhesion molecule-1
MMPs	matrix metalloproteinases
CT	computed tomography
MRI	magnetic resonance imaging
cIMT	carotid intimal and middle membrane thickness
XO	xanthine oxidase
CAT	catalase
GSH-Px	glutathione peroxidase

DOI: http://dx.doi.org/10.5772/intechopen.1009844

Author details

Qiyi Yu[1*†], Yidong Zhang[2†], Yifan Wu[3], Xianda Ma[1] and Yuxiao Chen[4]

1 Mellon College of Science, Carnegie Mellon University, Pittsburgh, USA

2 School of Pharmacy, Queen's University Belfast, Belfast, Northern Ireland

3 Mudi Meng Honors College, China Pharmaceutical University, Nanjing, China

4 Washington University School of Medicine in Saint Louis, Washington, USA

*Address all correspondence to: qiyiy@andrew.cmu.edu

† These authors contributed equally to the manuscript.

References

[1] Feigin VL, Stark BA, Johnson CO, Roth GA, Bisignano C, Abady GG, et al. Global, regional, and national burden of stroke and its risk factors, 1990-2019: A systematic analysis for the global burden of disease study 2019. The Lancet Neurology; 2021;**20**(10):795-820

[2] Delgado-Martín S, Martínez-Ruiz A. The role of ferroptosis as a regulator of oxidative stress in the pathogenesis of ischemic stroke. FEBS letters. 2024;**598**(17):2160-2173

[3] Rust R, Grönnert L, Weber RZ, Mulders G, Schwab ME. Refueling the ischemic CNS. Guidance molecules for vascular repair. Trends in Neurosciences. 2019;**42**(9):644-656

[4] Zhou M, Wang H, Zeng X, Yin P, Zhu J, Chen W, et al. Mortality, morbidity, and risk factors in China and its provinces, 1990-2017: A systematic analysis for the Global Burden of Disease Study 2017. Lancet (London, England). 2019;**394**(10204):1145-1158

[5] Zhou Y, Liao J, Mei Z, Liu X, Ge J. Insight into crosstalk between ferroptosis and necroptosis: Novel therapeutics in ischemic stroke. Oxidative Medicine and Cellular Longevity. 2021;**2021**:9991001. C-Editor: Zhao M; S-Editors: Yu J, Li CH; L-Editors: Yu J, Song LP; T-Editor: Jia Y

[6] Yousufuddin M, Young N. Aging and ischemic stroke. Aging. 2019;**11**(9):2542-2544

[7] Androvic P, Kirdajova D, Tureckova J, Zucha D, Rohlova E, Abaffy P, et al. Decoding the transcriptional response to ischemic stroke in young and aged mouse brain. Cell Reports. 2020;**31**(11):107777

[8] Fifield KE, Vanderluit JL. Rapid degeneration of neurons in the penumbra region following a small, focal ischemic stroke. The European Journal of Neuroscience. 2020;**52**(4):3196-3214

[9] Ghaffari A, Akbarfahimi M, Rostami HR. Discriminative factors for post-stroke depression. Asian Journal of Psychiatry. 2020;**48**:101863

[10] Love S. Oxidative stress in brain ischemia. Brain Pathology. 1999;**9**(1):119-131

[11] Wang X, Michaelis EK. Selective neuronal vulnerability to oxidative stress in the brain. Frontiers in Aging Neuroscience. 2010;**2**:1224

[12] Adibhatla RM, Hatcher JF. Lipid oxidation and peroxidation in CNS health and disease: From molecular mechanisms to therapeutic opportunities. Antioxidants & Redox Signaling. 2010;**12**(1):125-169

[13] Orellana-Urzúa S, Rojas I, Líbano L, Rodrigo R. Pathophysiology of ischemic stroke: Role of oxidative stress. Current Pharmaceutical Design. 2020;**26**(34):4246-4260

[14] Bladowski M, Gawrys J, Gajecki D, Szahidewicz-Krupska E, Sawicz-Bladowska A, Doroszko A. Role of the platelets and nitric oxide biotransformation in ischemic stroke: A translative review from bench to bedside. Oxidative Medicine and Cellular Longevity. 2020;**2020**(1):2979260

[15] Wu J, Jia J, Ji D, Jiao W, Huang Z, Zhang Y. Advances in nitric oxide regulators for the treatment of ischemic stroke. European Journal of Medicinal Chemistry. 2023;**262**:115912

[16] Wang Y, Hong F, Yang S. Roles of nitric oxide in brain ischemia and reperfusion. International Journal of Molecular Sciences. 2022;**23**(8):4243

[17] Lee H-M, Choi JW, Choi MS. Role of nitric oxide and protein S-nitrosylation in ischemia-reperfusion injury. Antioxidants. 2022;**11**(1):57

[18] Graff BJ, Payne SJ, El-Bouri WK. The ageing brain: Investigating the role of age in changes to the human cerebral microvasculature with an in silico model. Frontiers in Aging Neuroscience. 2021;**13**:632521

[19] Li Y, Choi WJ, Wei W, Song S, Zhang Q, Liu J, et al. Aging-associated changes in cerebral vasculature and blood flow as determined by quantitative optical coherence tomography angiography. Neurobiology of Aging. 2018;**70**:148-159

[20] Thomsen MS, Routhe LJ, Moos T. The vascular basement membrane in the healthy and pathological brain. Journal of Cerebral Blood Flow & Metabolism. 2017;**37**(10):3300-3317

[21] Ashorobi D, Ameer MA, Fernandez R. Thrombosis. In: StatPearls. Treasure Island (FL): StatPearls Publishing LLC.; 2024

[22] Rojsanga W, Sawanyawisuth K, Chotmongkol V, Tiamkao S, Kongbonkiat K, Kasemsap N. Clinical risk factors predictive of thrombotic stroke with large cerebral infarction. Neurology International. 2019;**11**(2):7941

[23] Bandera E, Botteri M, Minelli C, Sutton A, Abrams KR, Latronico N. Cerebral blood flow threshold of ischemic penumbra and infarct core in acute ischemic stroke. Stroke. 2006;**37**(5):1334-1339

[24] Graves SI, Baker DJ. Implicating endothelial cell senescence to dysfunction in the ageing and diseased brain. Basic & Clinical Pharmacology & Toxicology. 2020;**127**(2):102-110

[25] Li Z, Bi R, Sun S, Chen S, Chen J, Hu B, et al. The role of oxidative stress in acute ischemic stroke-related thrombosis. Oxidative Medicine and Cellular Longevity. 2022;**2022**(1):8418820

[26] Aries MJ, Elting JW, De Keyser J, Kremer BP, Vroomen PC. Cerebral autoregulation in stroke: A review of transcranial Doppler studies. Stroke. 2010;**41**(11):2697-2704

[27] Fan J-L, Brassard P, Rickards CA, Nogueira RC, Nasr N, McBryde FD, et al. Integrative cerebral blood flow regulation in ischemic stroke. Journal of Cerebral Blood Flow & Metabolism. 2022;**42**(3):387-403

[28] Singh V, Mishra VN, Chaurasia RN, Joshi D, Pandey V. Modes of calcium regulation in ischemic neuron. Indian Journal of Clinical Biochemistry: IJCB. 2019;**34**(3):246-253

[29] Liao QS, Du Q, Lou J, Xu JY, Xie R. Roles of Na(+)/Ca(2+) exchanger 1 in digestive system physiology and pathophysiology. World Journal of Gastroenterology. 2019;**25**(3):287-299

[30] Farooqui AA, Ong WY, Horrocks LA. Biochemical aspects of neurodegeneration in human brain: Involvement of neural membrane phospholipids and phospholipases A2. Neurochemical Research. 2004;**29**(11):1961-1977

[31] Ludhiadch A, Sharma R, Muriki A, Munshi A. Role of calcium homeostasis in ischemic stroke: A review. CNS & Neurological Disorders-Drug

Targets-CNS & Neurological Disorders;**21**(1):52-61

[32] Shehjar F, Maktabi B, Rahman ZA, Bahader GA, James AW, Naqvi A, et al. Stroke: Molecular mechanisms and therapies: Update on recent developments. Neurochemistry International. 2023;**162**:105458

[33] Wen B, Xu K, Huang R, Jiang T, Wang J, Chen J, et al. Preserving mitochondrial function by inhibiting GRP75 ameliorates neuron injury under ischemic stroke. Molecular Medicine Reports. 2022;**25**(5):165

[34] Bano D, Munarriz E, Chen HL, Ziviani E, Lippi G, Young KW, et al. The plasma membrane Na+/Ca2+ exchanger is cleaved by distinct protease families in neuronal cell death. Annals of the New York Academy of Sciences. 2007;**2007**:451-455

[35] Shen Z, Xiang M, Chen C, Ding F, Wang Y, Shang C, et al. Glutamate excitotoxicity: Potential therapeutic target for ischemic stroke. Biomedicine & Pharmacotherapy. 2022;**151**:113125

[36] Baltan S. Excitotoxicity and mitochondrial dysfunction underlie age-dependent ischemic white matter injury. In: Parpura V, Schousboe A, Verkhratsky A, editors. Glutamate and ATP at the Interface of Metabolism and Signaling in the Brain. Cham: Springer International Publishing; 2014. pp. 151-170

[37] Rice ME. H_2O_2: A dynamic neuromodulator. The Neuroscientist. 2011;**17**(4):389-406

[38] Manzanero S, Santro T, Arumugam TV. Neuronal oxidative stress in acute ischemic stroke: Sources and contribution to cell injury. Neurochemistry International. 2013;**62**(5):712-718

[39] Lesnefsky EJ, Hoppel CL. Oxidative phosphorylation and aging. Ageing Research Reviews. 2006;**5**(4):402-433

[40] Liu S, Shi H, Liu W, Furuichi T, Timmins GS, Liu KJ. Interstitial pO_2 in ischemic penumbra and core are differentially affected following transient focal cerebral ischemia in rats. Journal of Cerebral Blood Flow & Metabolism. 2004;**24**(3):343-349

[41] Hertz L. Bioenergetics of cerebral ischemia: A cellular perspective. Neuropharmacology. 2008;**55**(3):289-309

[42] Bryll A, Skrzypek J, Krzyściak W, Szelągowska M, Śmierciak N, Kozicz T, et al. Oxidative-antioxidant imbalance and impaired glucose metabolism in schizophrenia. Biomolecules. 2020;**10**(3):384

[43] Lewerenz J, Dargusch R, Maher P. Lactacidosis modulates glutathione metabolism and oxidative glutamate toxicity. Journal of Neurochemistry. 2010;**113**(2):502-514

[44] Radermacher KA, Wingler K, Kleikers P, Altenhöfer S, Hermans JR, Kleinschnitz C, et al. The 1027 th target candidate in stroke: Will NADPH oxidase hold up? Experimental & Translational Stroke Medicine. 2012;**4**:1-11

[45] Vallet P, Charnay Y, Steger K, Ogier-Denis E, Kovari E, Herrmann F, et al. Neuronal expression of the NADPH oxidase NOX4, and its regulation in mouse experimental brain ischemia. Neuroscience. 2005;**132**(2):233-238

[46] McCann SK, Dusting GJ, Roulston CL. Early increase of Nox4 NADPH oxidase and superoxide generation following endothelin-1-induced stroke in conscious rats. Journal of Neuroscience Research. 2008;**86**(11):2524-2534

[47] Sivandzade F, Prasad S, Bhalerao A, Cucullo L. NRF2 and NF-κB interplay in cerebrovascular and neurodegenerative disorders: Molecular mechanisms and possible therapeutic approaches. Redox Biology. 2019;**21**:101059

[48] Allen CL, Bayraktutan U. Oxidative stress and its role in the pathogenesis of Ischaemic stroke. International Journal of Stroke. 2009;**4**(6):461-470

[49] Tsubone TM, Martins WK, Franco MSF, Silva MN, Itri R, Baptista MS. Cellular compartments challenged by membrane photo-oxidation. Archives of Biochemistry and Biophysics. 2021;**697**:108665

[50] Kartha S. Leveraging Neuroinflammation Responses to Treat Pain Using Micellar Formulations Informed by Secretory Phospholipase A2 Responses in Neuropathy. Doctoral dissertation in University of Pennsylvania; 2021

[51] Trostchansky A, Wood I, Rubbo H. Regulation of arachidonic acid oxidation and metabolism by lipid electrophiles. Prostaglandins & Other Lipid Mediators. 2021;**152**:106482

[52] McCracken E, Valeriani V, Simpson C, Jover T, McCulloch J, Dewar D. The lipid peroxidationby-product4-hydroxynonenal is toxic to axons and oligodendrocytes. Journal of Cerebral Blood Flow and Metabolism: Official Journal of the International Society of Cerebral Blood Flow and Metabolism. 2000;**20**(11):1529-1536

[53] Matsuda S, Umeda M, Uchida H, Kato H, Araki T. Alterations of oxidative stress markers and apoptosis markers in the striatum after transient focal cerebral ischemia in rats. Journal of Neural Transmission (Vienna, Austria: 1996). 2009;**116**(4):395-404

[54] Barrera G, Pizzimenti S, Daga M, Dianzani C, Arcaro A, Cetrangolo GP, et al. Lipid peroxidation-derived aldehydes, 4-hydroxynonenal and malondialdehyde in aging-related disorders. Antioxidants. 2018;**7**(8):102

[55] Chen S, Li Q, Shi H, Li F, Duan Y, Guo Q. New insights into the role of mitochondrial dynamics in oxidative stress-induced diseases. Biomedicine & Pharmacotherapy. 2024;**178**:117084

[56] Oke O, Akosile O, Oni A, Opowoye I, Ishola C, Adebiyi J, et al. Oxidative stress in poultry production. Poultry Science 2024:104003

[57] Ahmad S, Khan H, Rafi Z, Shahab U, Ashraf JM, Ahmad MK, et al. Free radicals and their relation to diseases and protection against them. Clinical Applications of Biomolecules in Disease Diagnosis: A Comprehensive Guide to Biochemistry and Metabolism. Springer; 2024. pp. 323-350

[58] Saki M, Prakash A. DNA damage related crosstalk between the nucleus and mitochondria. Free Radical Biology and Medicine. 2017;**107**:216-227

[59] Kowalska M, Piekut T, Prendecki M, Sodel A, Kozubski W, Dorszewska J. Mitochondrial and nuclear DNA oxidative damage in physiological and pathological aging. DNA and Cell Biology. 2020;**39**(8):1410-1420

[60] Yazğan B, Yazğan Y, Övey İS, Nazıroğlu M. Raloxifene and tamoxifen reduce PARP activity, cytokine and oxidative stress levels in the brain and blood of ovariectomized rats. Journal of Molecular Neuroscience: MN. 2016;**60**(2):214-222

[61] Veenman L. Raloxifene as treatment for various types of brain injuries and neurodegenerative diseases: A good

start. International Journal of Molecular Sciences. 2020;**21**(20):7586

[62] Zhou Z, Arroum T, Luo X, Kang R, Lee YJ, Tang D, et al. Diverse functions of cytochrome c in cell death and disease. Cell Death and Differentiation. 2024;**31**(4):387-404

[63] Kim GW, Sugawara T, Chan PH. Involvement of oxidative stress and caspase-3 in cortical infarction after photothrombotic ischemia in mice. Journal of Cerebral Blood Flow and Metabolism: Official Journal of the International Society of Cerebral Blood Flow and Metabolism. 2000;**20**(12):1690-1701

[64] Shadfar S, Brocardo M, Atkin JD. The complex mechanisms by which neurons die following DNA damage in neurodegenerative diseases. International Journal of Molecular Sciences. 2022;**23**(5):2484

[65] Qz T, St Z, Lei P. Mechanisms of neuronal cell death in ischemic stroke and their therapeutic implications. Medicinal Research Reviews. 2022;**42**(1):259-305

[66] Yu J, Zhang L. PUMA, a potent killer with or without p53. Oncogene. 2008;**27**(1):S71-S83

[67] Li X-Q, Yu Q, Chen F-S, Tan W-F, Zhang Z-L, Ma H. Inhibiting aberrant p53-PUMA feedback loop activation attenuates ischaemia reperfusion-induced neuroapoptosis and neuroinflammation in rats by downregulating caspase 3 and the NF-κB cytokine pathway. Journal of Neuroinflammation. 2018;**15**:1-13

[68] Sugawara T, Fujimura M, Noshita N, Kim GW, Saito A, Hayashi T, et al. Neuronal death/survival signaling pathways in cerebral ischemia. NeuroRx: The Journal of the American Society for Experimental NeuroTherapeutics. 2004;**1**(1):17-25

[69] Suzuki Y, Enokido Y, Yamada K, Inaba M, Kuwata K, Hanada N, et al. The effect of rapamycin, NVP-BEZ235, aspirin, and metformin on PI3K/AKT/mTOR signaling pathway of PIK3CA-related overgrowth spectrum (PROS). Oncotarget. 2017;**8**(28):45470

[70] Lingappan K. NF-κB in oxidative stress. Current Opinion in Toxicology. 2018;**7**:81-86

[71] Xu G, Dong F, Su L, Tan Z-X, Lei M, Li L, et al. The role and therapeutic potential of nuclear factor κB (NF-κB) in ischemic stroke. Biomedicine & Pharmacotherapy. 2024;**171**:116140

[72] Wu Y-F, Jin K-Y, Wang D-P, Lin Q, Sun J, Su S-H, et al. VEGF loaded nanofiber membranes inhibit chronic cerebral hypoperfusion-induced cognitive dysfunction by promoting HIF-1a/VEGF mediated angiogenesis. Nanomedicine: Nanotechnology, Biology and Medicine. 2023;**48**:102639

[73] Szyller J, Bil-Lula I. Heat shock proteins in oxidative stress and ischemia/reperfusion injury and benefits from physical exercises: A review to the current knowledge. Oxidative Medicine and Cellular Longevity. 2021;**2021**(1):6678457

[74] Chen XM, Chen HS, Xu MJ, Shen JG. Targeting reactive nitrogen species: A promising therapeutic strategy for cerebral ischemia-reperfusion injury. Acta Pharmacologica Sinica. 2013;**34**(1):67-77

[75] Jurcau A, Simion A. Oxidative stress in the pathogenesis of Alzheimer's disease and cerebrovascular disease with therapeutic implications. CNS &

Neurological Disorders Drug Targets. 2020;**19**(2):94-108

[76] Huang Z, Huang PL, Ma J, Meng W, Ayata C, Fishman MC, et al. Enlarged infarcts in endothelial nitric oxide synthase knockout mice are attenuated by nitro-L-arginine. Journal of Cerebral Blood Flow and Metabolism: Official Journal of the International Society of Cerebral Blood Flow and Metabolism. 1996;**16**(5):981-987

[77] Danielisova V, Burda J, Nemethova M, GottliebM.Aminoguanidineadministration ameliorates hippocampal damage after middle cerebral artery occlusion in rat. Neurochemical Research. 2011;**36**:476-486

[78] Chen Z-q, Mou R-t, Feng D-x, Wang Z, Chen G. The role of nitric oxide in stroke. Medical Gas Research. 2017;**7**(3):194-203

[79] Pannu R, Singh I. Pharmacological strategies for the regulation of inducible nitric oxide synthase: Neurodegenerative versus neuroprotective mechanisms. Neurochemistry International. 2006;**49**(2):170-182

[80] Iadecola C, Zhang F, Casey R, Nagayama M, Ross ME. Delayed reduction of ischemic brain injury and neurological deficits in mice lacking the inducible nitric oxide synthase gene. The Journal of Neuroscience: The Official Journal of the Society for Neuroscience. 1997;**17**(23):9157-9164

[81] Ferriero DM, Holtzman DM, Black SM, Sheldon RA. Neonatal mice lacking neuronal nitric oxide synthase are less vulnerable to hypoxic-ischemic injury. Neurobiology of Disease. 1996;**3**(1):64-71

[82] Marín-Ramos NI, Chen TC. Chapter Three The blood brain barrier: Molecular and cellular function. Advances in Brain Vascular Research. 2020. p. 48

[83] Chang DI, Hosomi N, Lucero J, Heo JH, Abumiya T, Mazar AP, et al. Activation systems for latent matrix metalloproteinase-2 are upregulated immediately after focal cerebral ischemia. Journal of Cerebral Blood Flow and Metabolism: Official Journal of the International Society of Cerebral Blood Flow and Metabolism. 2003;**23**(12):1408-1419

[84] Rosenberg GA, Yang Y. Vasogenic edema due to tight junction disruption by matrix metalloproteinases in cerebral ischemia. Neurosurgical Focus. 2007;**22**(5):E4

[85] Gu Y, Zheng G, Xu M, Li Y, Chen X, Zhu W, et al. Caveolin-1 regulates nitric oxide-mediated matrix metalloproteinases activity and blood–brain barrier permeability in focal cerebral ischemia and reperfusion injury. Journal of Neurochemistry. 2012;**120**(1):147-156

[86] Moro MA, Almeida A, Bolaños JP, Lizasoain I. Mitochondrial respiratory chain and free radical generation in stroke. Free Radical Biology & Medicine. 2005;**39**(10):1291-1304

[87] Garry PS, Ezra M, Rowland MJ, Westbrook J, Pattinson KT. The role of the nitric oxide pathway in brain injury and its treatment—From bench to bedside. Experimental Neurology. 2015;**263**:235-243

[88] Ames BN, Shigenaga MK, Hagen TM. Oxidants, antioxidants, and the degenerative diseases of aging. Proceedings of the National Academy of Sciences of the United States of America. 1993;**90**(17):7915-7922

[89] Floyd RA, Hensley K. Oxidative stress in brain aging: Implications for

therapeutics of neurodegenerative diseases. Neurobiology of Aging. 2002;**23**(5):795-807

[90] Bettio LE, Rajendran L, Gil-Mohapel J. The effects of aging in the hippocampus and cognitive decline. Neuroscience & Biobehavioral Reviews. 2017;**79**:66-86

[91] Wu Z, Yu J, Zhu A, Nakanishi H. Nutrients, microglia aging, and brain aging. Oxidative Medicine and Cellular Longevity. 2016;**2016**:7498528

[92] Mattson MP, Arumugam TV. Hallmarks of brain aging: Adaptive and pathological modification by metabolic states. Cell Metabolism. 2018;**27**(6):1176-1199

[93] Ham PB 3rd, Raju R. Mitochondrial function in hypoxic ischemic injury and influence of aging. Progress in Neurobiology. 2017;**157**:92-116

[94] Rzechorzek W, Zhang H, Buckley BK, Hua K, Pomp D, Faber JE. Aerobic exercise prevents rarefaction of pial collaterals and increased stroke severity that occur with aging. Journal of Cerebral Blood Flow & Metabolism. 2017;**37**(11):3544-3555

[95] Xie Q, Peng S, Tao L, Ruan H, Yang Y, Li T-M, et al. E2F transcription factor 1 regulates cellular and organismal senescence by inhibiting Forkhead box O transcription factors. Journal of Biological Chemistry. 2014;**289**(49):34205-34213

[96] Shao A, Lin D, Wang L, Tu S, Lenahan C, Zhang J. Oxidative stress at the crossroads of aging, stroke and depression. Aging and Disease. 2020;**11**(6):1537-1566

[97] Khatri R, Vellipuram AR, Maud A, Cruz-Flores S, Rodriguez GJ. Current endovascular approach to the management of acute ischemic stroke. Current Cardiology Reports. 2018;**20**(6):46

[98] Chugh C. Acute ischemic stroke: Management approach. Indian Journal of Critical Care Medicine: Peer-Reviewed, Official Publication of Indian Society of Critical Care Medicine. 2019;**23** (Suppl. 2):S140-S146

[99] Kumar V, Bishayee K, Park S, Lee U, Kim J. Oxidative stress in cerebrovascular disease and associated diseases. Frontiers in Endocrinology. 2023;**14**:1124419

[100] Rosskopf J, Kloth C, Dreyhaupt J, Braun M, Schmitz BL, Graeter T. Thin slices and maximum intensity projection reconstructions increase sensitivity to hyperdense middle cerebral artery sign in acute ischemic stroke. Cerebrovascular Diseases (Basel, Switzerland). 2020;**49**(4):437-441

[101] Radhiana H, Syazarina SO, Shahizon Azura MM, Hilwati H, Sobri MA. Non-contrast computed tomography in acute ischaemic stroke: A pictorial review. The Medical Journal of Malaysia. 2013;**68**(1):93-100

[102] Rimmele DL, Thomalla G. Wake-up stroke: Clinical characteristics, imaging findings, and treatment option—An update. Frontiers in Neurology. 2014;**5**:35

[103] Montaner J. Stroke biomarkers: Can they help us to guide stroke thrombolysis? Drug News & Perspectives. 2006;**19**(9):523-532

[104] Bsat S, Halaoui A, Kobeissy F, Moussalem C, El Houshiemy MN, Kawtharani S, et al. Acute ischemic stroke biomarkers: A new era with diagnostic promise? Acute Medicine & Surgery. 2021;**8**(1):e696

[105] Boehme AK, Esenwa C, Elkind MS. Stroke risk factors, genetics, and

prevention. Circulation Research. 2017;**120**(3):472-495

[106] Alexandrov AV, Grotta JC. Arterial reocclusion in stroke patients treated with intravenous tissue plasminogen activator. Neurology. 2002;**59**(6):862-867

[107] Elsayed WM, Abdel-Gawad E-HA, Mesallam DI, El-Serafy TS. The relationship between oxidative stress and acute ischemic stroke severity and functional outcome. The Egyptian Journal of Neurology, Psychiatry and Neurosurgery. 2020;**56**:1-6

[108] Popiela TJ, Krzyściak W, Pilato F, Ligęzka A, Bystrowska B, Bukowska-Strakova K, et al. The assessment of endovascular therapies in ischemic stroke: management, problems and future approaches. Journal of Clinical Medicine. 2022;**11**(7):1864

[109] Pawluk H, Kołodziejska R, Grześk G, Woźniak A, Kozakiewicz M, Kosinska A, et al. Increased oxidative stress markers in acute ischemic stroke patients treated with thrombolytics. International Journal of Molecular Sciences. 2022;**23**(24):15625

[110] Menon B, Ramalingam K, Kumar R. Evaluating the role of oxidative stress in acute ischemic stroke. Journal of Neurosciences in Rural Practice. 2020;**11**(01):156-159

[111] Kamal FZ, Lefter R, Jaber H, Balmus I-M, Ciobica A, Iordache A-C. The role of potential oxidative biomarkers in the prognosis of acute ischemic stroke and the exploration of antioxidants as possible preventive and treatment options. International Journal of Molecular Sciences. 2023;**24**(7):6389

[112] Wang J, Gao S, Lenahan C, Gu Y, Wang X, Fang Y, et al. Melatonin as an antioxidant agent in stroke: An updated review. Aging and Disease. 2022;**13**(6):1823

[113] Wang A, Yang Y, Su Z, Yue W, Hao H, Ren L, et al. Association of oxidized low-density lipoprotein with prognosis of stroke and stroke subtypes. Stroke. 2017;**48**(1):91-97

[114] Yu Q, Zhang Y, Zhang Y, Zhang W. Diagnostic genes identification and molecular classification patterns based on oxidative stress-related genes in ischemic stroke. International Conference on Medical Imaging and Computer-Aided Diagnosis: 2023. Springer; 2023. pp. 179-199

[115] Plubell DL, Fenton AM, Rosario S, Bergstrom P, Wilmarth PA, Clark WM, et al. High-density lipoprotein carries markers that track with recovery from stroke. Circulation Research. 2020;**127**(10):1274-1287

[116] Jelinek M, Jurajda M, Duris K. Oxidative stress in the brain: Basic concepts and treatment strategies in stroke. Antioxidants. 2021;**10**(12):1886

[117] Margaill I, Plotkine M, Lerouet D. Antioxidant strategies in the treatment of stroke. Free Radical Biology and Medicine. 2005;**39**(4):429-443

[118] Genovese T, Mazzon E, Paterniti I, Esposito E, Bramanti P, Cuzzocrea S. Modulation of NADPH oxidase activation in cerebral ischemia/reperfusion injury in rats. Brain Research. 2011;**1372**:92-102

[119] Tang L, Ye K, Yang X, Zheng J. Apocynin attenuates cerebral infarction after transient focal ischaemia in rats. Journal of International Medical Research. 2007;**35**(4):517-522

[120] Touyz RM. Apocynin, NADPH oxidase, and vascular cells: A complex matter. Hypertension. 2008;**51**:172-174

[121] Heumüller S, Wind S, Barbosa-Sicard E, Schmidt HHHW, Busse R, Schröder K, et al. Apocynin is not an inhibitor of vascular NADPH oxidases but an antioxidant. Hypertension. 2008;**51**(2):211-217

[122] Kleinschnitz C, Grund H, Wingler K, Armitage ME, Jones E, Mittal M, et al. Post-stroke inhibition of induced NADPH oxidase type 4 prevents oxidative stress and neurodegeneration. PLoS biology. 2010;**8**(9):e1000479

[123] Furuhashi M. New insights into purine metabolism in metabolic diseases: Role of xanthine oxidoreductase activity. American Journal of Physiology-Endocrinology and Metabolism. 2020;**319**(5):E827-E834

[124] Schlesinger N, Brunetti L. Beyond urate lowering: Analgesic and anti-inflammatory properties of allopurinol. Seminars in Arthritis and Rheumatism: 2020. Elsevier; 2020. pp. 444-450

[125] Luo J, Yan D, Li S, Liu S, Zeng F, Cheung CW, et al. Allopurinol reduces oxidative stress and activates Nrf2/p62 to attenuate diabetic cardiomyopathy in rats. Journal of Cellular and Molecular Medicine. 2020;**24**(2):1760-1773

[126] Yamashita T, Abe K. Update on antioxidant therapy with edaravone: Expanding applications in neurodegenerative diseases. International Journal of Molecular Sciences. 2024;**25**(5):2945

[127] White BC, Sullivan JM, DeGracia DJ, O'Neil BJ, Neumar RW, Grossman LI, et al. Brain ischemia and reperfusion: Molecular mechanisms of neuronal injury. Journal of the Neurological Sciences. 2000;**179**(S1-2):1-33

[128] Nakagawa H, Ohyama R, Kimata A, Suzuki T, Miyata N. Hydroxyl radical scavenging by edaravone derivatives: Efficient scavenging by 3-methyl-1-(pyridin-2-yl)-5-pyrazolone with an intramolecular base. Bioorganic & Medicinal Chemistry Letters. 2006;**16**(23):5939-5942

[129] Edaravone Acute Infarction Study Group. Effect of a novel free radical scavenger, edaravone (MCI-186), on acute brain infarction. Randomized, placebo-controlled, double-blind study at multicenters. Cerebrovascular Diseases (Basel, Switzerland). 2003;**15**(3):222-229

[130] Rodrigo R, Fernandez-Gajardo R, Gutiérrez R, Manuel Matamala J, Carrasco R, Miranda-Merchak A, et al. Oxidative stress and pathophysiology of ischemic stroke: Novel therapeutic opportunities. CNS & Neurological Disorders-Drug Targets (Formerly Current Drug Targets-CNS & Neurological Disorders). 2013;**12**(5):698-714

[131] Morelli MB, Gambardella J, Castellanos V, Trimarco V, Santulli G. Vitamin C and cardiovascular disease: An update. Antioxidants. 2020;**9**(12):1227

[132] Fujimura M, Morita-Fujimura Y, Noshita N, Sugawara T, Kawase M, Chan PH. The cytosolic antioxidant copper/zinc-superoxide dismutase prevents the early release of mitochondrial cytochrome c in ischemic brain after transient focal cerebral ischemia in mice. Journal of Neuroscience. 2000;**20**(8):2817-2824

[133] Sugawara T, Lewén A, Gasche Y, Yu F, Chan PH. Overexpression of SOD1 protects vulnerable motor neurons after spinal cord injury by attenuating mitochondrial cytochrome c release. The FASEB Journal. 2002;**16**(14):1997-1999

[134] Shirley R, Ord EN, Work LM. Oxidative stress and the use of

antioxidants in stroke. Antioxidants. 2014;**3**(3):472-501

[135] Diener HC. Multinational randomised controlled trial of lubeluzole in acute ischaemic stroke. Cerebrovascular Diseases. 1998;**8**(3):172-181

[136] Niatsetskaya ZV, Sosunov SA, Matsiukevich D, Utkina-Sosunova IV, Ratner VI, Starkov AA, et al. The oxygen free radicals originating from mitochondrial complex I contribute to oxidative brain injury following hypoxia–ischemia in neonatal mice. Journal of Neuroscience. 2012;**32**(9):3235-3244

[137] Murphy MP. Antioxidants as therapies: Can we improve on nature? Free Radical Biology and Medicine. 2014;**66**:20-23

[138] Fock EM, Parnova RG. Protective effect of mitochondria-targeted antioxidants against inflammatory response to lipopolysaccharide challenge: A review. Pharmaceutics. 2021;**13**(2):144

Chapter 3

Theoretical Aspects of Protein Aggregation and Neurodegenerative Diseases

Vishal Singh and Priya Dey

Abstract

The polypeptide chain folds spontaneously into a native state to do function correctly. However, phenotypic and genotypic variations may induce abnormal amino acid modifications in the protein sequence and lead to misfolding that disrupts normal cellular function. The protein quality control system present in the cell manages the misfolded proteins and helps them to either refold back to their native state or degrade them to amino acids and eventually replace them with newly synthesized replicas. This phenomenon, known as protein turnover, is highly specific and precisely regulated process that involves a constant renewal of the functional proteins by allowing the damaged or non-functional ones to be eliminated. Factors such as aging, genetic mutation, oxidative stress, pH, and temperature result in failure of the protein turnover process that leads to the formation of aggregates/fibrils through self-association of the misfolded proteins. Typically, these aggregates are highly organized hydrogen-bonded structures that are more stable compared to the native protein. A wide variety of debilitating disorders such as Alzheimer's, Parkinson's, amyotrophic lateral sclerosis, Huntington's, and dementia are directly linked with the deposition of aggregates in the cells. Understanding the theoretical aspects of protein aggregation provides a foundation for developing therapeutic strategies of preventing these neurodegenerative disorders.

Keywords: protein quality control, protein turnover, protein misfolding and aggregation, neurodegenerative disorders, free energy landscape, intrinsically disordered proteins

1. Introduction

Proteins are highly complex and most versatile macromolecules which play a crucial role in all living organisms. Proteins are composed of 22 naturally occurring amino acids, which are covalently linked through peptide bonds. The size of protein varies from small peptides with tens of amino acids to large ones with thousands of amino acids, and thus, different proteins exhibit varying amino acid sequences. Most cellular functions are fulfilled or regulated by proteins. Proteins perform a diverse range of functions within and outside the cell and serve a key role in all biological processes. Proteins catalyze essential biochemical reactions, act as messengers to transmit physical and chemical information between cells, tissues, and organs, help the tissues for growth and maintenance, transport and store nutrients like vitamins, minerals, oxygen,and blood sugar, strengthen human health by forming antibodies and provide the structure and strength to the body [1–4]. Proteins also help in maintaining the fluid balance by keeping water in the blood and waste cleanup by eliminating aberrant proteins [1, 5].

2. Folding of protein

The newly synthesized unfolded polypeptide chain or random coil lacks any stable conformation as it has high energy and high entropy. This linear chain of amino acids interacts with each other, which may help to fold the chain into a well-defined three-dimensional (3*D*) structure, known as the native state. The hydrophobic effect is an important driving force behind the folding processes that allow the hydrophobic residue to find in the internal core of the 3*D* conformation with minimum or no contact with water [6–8]. Therefore, these hydrophobic interactions have an impact on the primary structure of protein and then lead to the formation of secondary and tertiary structures. Intramolecular H-bonds, disulfide bond, and ionic interactions also assist toward the stability of the tertiary structure of a protein. Thus, the folding process is completely a physical process where the polypeptide chain finds its unique correct 3*D* structure, which is essential to function and have minimum energy with minimum entropy. Thus, protein folding is essential for a polypeptide chain to acquire its proper 3*D* structure and function. Levinthal suggested that it is impossible to choose the native state of any protein from its astronomical number of possible conformations through the random search method as it takes more than the age of universe, that is, millions of years [9, 10]. But in reality, the protein folds in the biological time scale of a microsecond to millisecond [11–16]. This indicates that the protein search its native state through a definite pathway directed toward only one minimum energy conformation, known as globule minima, where the protein is thermodynamically stable and kinetically accessible at the same temperature [17–19].

The thermodynamic stability of a protein is given through the change in folding free energy, ΔG, as

$$\Delta G = \Delta H - T\Delta S \tag{1}$$

here, H and S are the enthalpy and the entropy of the protein, respectively, and T is the absolute temperature of the system. During the folding process, the entropy of the protein decreases, so the entropic term "$-T\Delta S$" becomes positive but at the same time interaction like hydrophobic interaction, H-bonding and van dar Wall forces release some amount of heat, so the enthalpic term "ΔH" becomes negative. When the enthalpic term dominates over the entropic term, the overall "ΔG" becomes negative. Thus, we can say that the protein folding is a spontaneous process. But due to change in environmental conditions like T, P, pH and mutation in the polypeptide chain protein fails to fold and gets trapped in some other configuration and loses its functions.

3. Protein misfolding and aggregation

Now it is clear that the folded state of protein is sampled through stochastic search method rather than random sampling of all the possible configurations [20–22]. The folding process relies on the correct interaction of the residues of protein, which are closer to each other during conformational fluctuation, these interaction is called as native contacts. This folding process is complex and involves the formation of secondary structure such as α-helix and β-sheet. This is also mediated by various suitable interactions like H-bonding, hydrophobic and electrostatic interactions and Van der Waals forces [23, 24]. The folded protein directed toward minimum energy conformation as it is more stable than the near-native/non-native conformations, which consist of non-native contacts. These near-native conformations may be considered as aberrant or misfolded proteins. Thus, the folding is essential for function as the quality control mechanism ensures the correct folding of the polypeptide chain [22, 25–28]. Depending on the efficiency of this quality control mechanism, these aberrant or misfolded proteins may be eliminated from the system or/and stabilized through the formation of aggregates (refer to **Figure 1**). However, folding pathways may be disrupted by the abnormal changes in the amino acid sequences, which leads to the formation of misfolded protein that have capability to self-associate to form aggregates. Also, variation in the cellular environment such as temperature, pH, oxidative stress etc. and any type of mutation in the DNA sequence with aging may reduce the efficiency of quality control mechanism, resulting the alteration in the folding process, which is responsible for protein misfolding/aggregation [30–34]. The deposition of these misfolded/aggregates in the brain is directly related to neurodegenerative disorders (NDDs) that include multiple non-communicable age-related diseases such as Alzheimer's disease (AD), Parkinson's disease (PD), Amyotrophic lateral sclerosis (ALS), Huntington's disease (HD), Creutzfeldt-Jakob disease, Prion disease, and many more [32, 35–39].

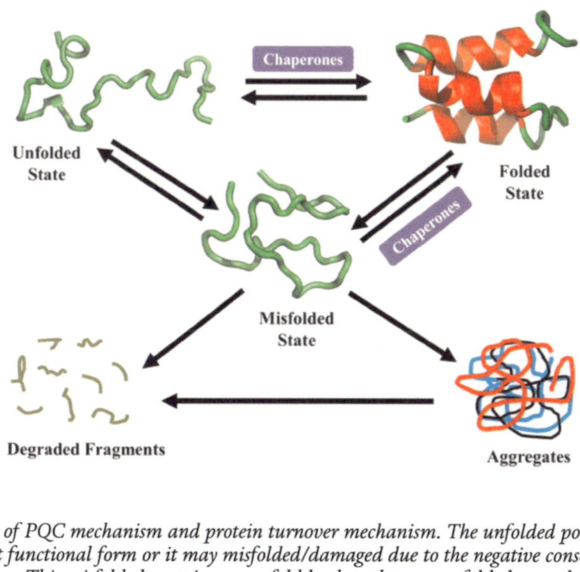

Figure 1.
A schematic diagram of PQC mechanism and protein turnover mechanism. The unfolded polypeptide chain may be folded to its correct functional form or it may misfolded/damaged due to the negative consequences of cell environment and aging. This misfolded protein may refold back to the correct folded state through chaperones (PQC mechanism) or it being degraded, and a new replica of the polypeptide chain is synthesized (protein turnover). Misfolded protein may self-associate to form an aggregate as the PQC mechanism fails. This process is practically irreversible as aggregates are more stable (adapted from Singh [29]).

3.1 Protein quality control

Low temperature and low concentration are essential for protein folding in the test tube experiments but in cellular environment, protein folding takes place in a complex cellular environment with very high concentration and at comparatively high temperature at 37°C or even high during fever [22, 40]. With this, polypeptide chains are committed to the correct folding even with the change in the cellular environment. However, physical and chemical stress may harm the protein structure and disturb the folding process that may lead to the misfolding of the protein [41–43]. Misfolding can also occur through mutation/error in the primary structure of the protein, which changes its ability to fold properly [44]. In this way, the misfolding or aberrant proteins are regularly produced in the cell. Therefore, to assist the efficiency of the folding process in the complex cellular environment and to protect from the negative consequences of environmental changes, the protein quality control (PQC) system evolves in the cell in such a way that eliminates the damaged polypeptide chain and the misfolded protein and guide the folding process to counteract aggregation and toxic effect. This process is mainly assisted by the molecular chaperones, which generally direct the aberrant protein to either refold back to the system or remove it from the system before it exerts a toxic effect [22, 34], as shown in **Figure 1**. The folding intermediate or non/near-native protein may bind with the chapreone at active side in such a way that it again come to the normal folding process. The binding sites of chaperones also capture the exposed hydrophobic region of amino acids in misfolded, unfolded and/or partially folded proteins and thus protect them against aggregation during the folding of polypeptide chain [26, 44, 45, 46]. The misfolded or damaged protein that escapes the PQC system may self-associate to form aggregates.

Different chaperones are used for different folding processes depending on their partially folded or non-native conformations. Heat shock proteins (HSPs) majorly belong to molecular chaperones because they are prompted by different stresses like oxidative stress, heat shock, and toxic chemical [47, 48]. The subunit of different sizes of HSPs like Hsp40, Hsp60, Hsp70, and Hsp90 work as molecular chaperones [48]. Some chaperones like Hsp110 work for different folding intermediates while other

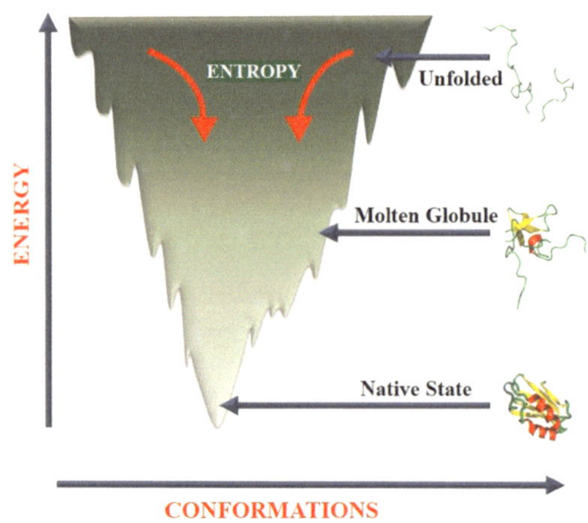

Figure 2.
A schematic diagram of the rugged free energy landscape where the native state is found at the global minimum of this landscape.

chaperones like Hsp70 and Hsp60 perform several functions. On the basis of their mode of action, they are classified into three distinct categories as.

i. *Unfolding chaperones*: This class of chaperones (Hsp70 and Hsp60s) is able to bind with misfolded proteins and unfold them either to start a new folding process or degradation [49, 50].

ii. *Folding chaperones*: Some chaperones like human Hsp70 and yeast Hsp104 in complex with Hsp40 and Hsp110 forcefully unfold the aggregates into a natively folded state. This type of chaperones acts as "disaggregates" that use the energy of ATP hydrolysis for function [27, 51, 52].

iii. *Holding chaperones*: Most molecular chaperones such as Hsp70 hold the protein at the unfolded state and pass them to the folding chaperones for proper folding [53, 54].

The central task of PQC system includes the maintenance of the functional proteins and constant turnover of proteins by removal of the misfolded/damaged proteins from the cellular system. Though under the normal condition, PQC system is highly dynamic, due to the overload of misfolded proteins, gene variation, negative consequences of environment, and aging, the efficiency of PQC system decreases, triggering the onset of diseases.

3.2 Protein turnover

The efficiency of quality control mechanism is reduced with aging as the cellular environment may change due to oxidative stress, mutation/error, and other negative consequences. Therefore, aging, a complex phenomenon, plays a main role in the biological process at different stages and eventually loses the function of protein in the cell [55]. Thus, cells do not maintain proper protein homeostasis due to the degradation of the proteins that cause age-related diseases. Protein turnover re-establishes the balance between degradation and the synthesis of proteins [12, 56]. Proteins inside the cell are degraded at continuous intervals and insistently replaced with new replicas of these proteins [55]. This turnover process is certain and controlled (highly specific and precisely regulated) and involves continuous production of newly synthesized functional proteins by allowing the aberrant/damaged or non-functional ones to be eliminated from the cell cycle [57, 58]. The turnover rate depends on the half-life of the protein; therefore, it is different for the different proteins. The half-life varies from a few seconds to several days in the cell [55, 57, 59, 60]. Some studies [55, 60, 61] confirm that the half-life of proteins is 0.5–35 hours in dividing mammalian cells and $\sim$43 hours in non-dividing cells.

4. Free energy landscape

According to Levinthal, it is impossible to search the native conformation for the polypeptide chain as it has an astronomical large number of conformations [9]. To overcome this issue, several experimental and theoretical studies [62–64] show that this paradox may be settled through the calculation of the free energy of each and every conformation. The plot of free energy versus conformational space indicates the conformations from lower energy to the higher energy, and it is directed toward the lower energy. The minimum energy conformation is known as native conformation, and this diagram is particularly known as free energy landscape (FEL). In this funnel shape of landscape, the free energy and the entropy of the system continuously decrease, and the process is spontaneous. For this case, enthalpy plays a major role in keeping the "ΔG" negative, this explanation is given in the above Section "Folding of Protein." The landscape of the folding processes particularly provides the stochastic description of the kinetics of folding, misfolding and aggregation processes.

The funnel shape landscape is result of the formation of several favorable/native interactions (intramolecular) between amino acid residues which mostly help the chain to find their functional form. The energy landscape theory describes the minimum and maximum energy conformations as well as multiple distinct pathways having several local and near-native energy conformations which is directed toward native state or the global minimum of the landscape as the polypeptide chain always searches the a lower energy conformation over the higher one [23, 43]. These lower energy conformations are well separated from the higher one through the energy barriers [17, 65–68]. The naturally occurring small proteins directly approach the native state as it synthesized and also have the tendency to overcome the energy barrier to reach the folded state [11, 18, 65, 69, 70]. Therefore, such protein have smooth type of funnel which shows the relatively fast folding due to evolutionary selection of the sequences and having less number of conformations. In other ways, larger protein may have relatively large number of conformations that may get trapped in some other conformation having local minima energy, this state is commonly known as the molten globule state [71–73]. The energy barrier for this case may be relatively high, so for the chain, it is difficult to cross this potential barrier to reach the minimum energy conformation [74]. Sometimes, specific molecular chaperons may help these polypeptide chains to cross the barrier and reach their native or minimum energy state [75]. This type of landscape is particularly known as a rugged funnel-shaped energy landscape, which shows on and off pathways to the folded/native state of the protein. The rugged funnel shape free energy landscape is shown in **Figure 2**. The pathway of protein on the free energy landscape depends on their physicochemical condition and the structural feature of the polypeptide chain. The folding process of the polypeptide chain to its correct functional form is based on the single chain with intramolecular interactions.

However, any genotypic and phenotypic changes in the polypeptide chain may change the interaction between the amino acids residues, which changes the conformational space and the free energies of the polypeptide chain that consequently alter their surface of the free energy landscape [22, 76]. The change in the landscape consists of the formation of new local minima or different stable states, which do not correspond to the global minima or the native state of protein [22, 76]. Also, it is not necessary for the polypeptide chain to cross the potential barrier that is trapped in other conformations and reach the correct folded state even if the molecular chaperons may assist in their folding process. In this case, the protein is trapped in the new local minima, which is defined as the misfolded or partially folded protein. Usually, this type of protein consists of high β-sheet propensity and has low mean net charge due to the exposed region of the hydrophobic residues [28, 77–79]. Eventually, these misfolded or partially folded proteins may self-associate to form an aggregate and lead to several neurodegenerative diseases. Here, the self-association of the misfolded/partially folded proteins consists of the different folding processes of the same polypeptide chain that may connected through the intermolecular interactions. The kinetic battle between intramolecular (for native folding) and intermolecular interactions (for the self-association of the misfolded protein to form an aggregate) may increase the ruggedness of the energy landscape [80]. This dramatic nature of the landscape is due to external factors like changes in environmental conditions (such as pH, temperature, and pressure), high protein concentration in the cell, etc. [80, 81]. The aggregates are kinetically trapped in the lowest basin of the free energy landscape, and hence, they indicate an extremely stable state as compared to the native state. Hence, the native state does not always correspond to the minimum energy conformation, and aggregates are even more stable than the native state. The formation of different types of aggregates such as amorphous aggregates and amyloid fibrils increases the ruggedness of the landscape. **Figure 3** shows the free energy landscape of folding, misfolding, and aggregation of the polypeptide chain. This landscape has two sides; one consists of the folding process of the native state, that is, intramolecular interaction, and the other one denotes the aggregation side of the landscape, that is, intermolecular interaction. In the aggregation side of landscape, high-energy and high-entropy regions consist of monomers and oligomers, while low-energy and low entropy regions represent two distinct states of aggregates i.e. amorphous and amyloid fibrils [45, 82]. This suggests that at high concentration of protein, amyloid fibrils are more generic and thermodynamically the most stable structures.

However, the shape of the landscape is not always be the rugged funnel shape that directed toward lower energy conformation either native or the aggregates. For some polypeptide chain the energy of all the possible conformation is found to be similar. This happens mostly for the case of intrinsically disordered proteins (IDPs). The energy landscape of an intrinsically disordered protein refers to the distribution of energy states that the protein may occupy. Unlike structured proteins with well-defined 3D conformations, intrinsically disordered proteins do not have a fixed conformation and, instead,

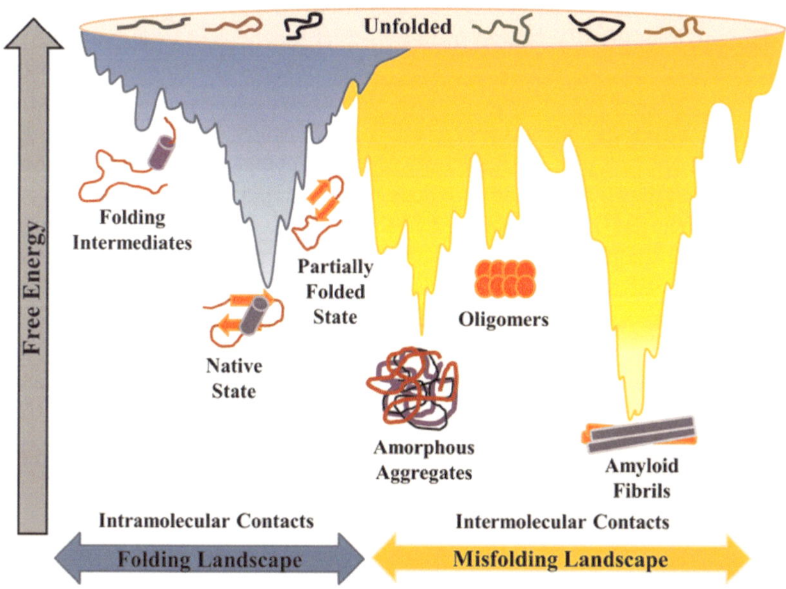

Figure 3.
A schematic representation of a combined free energy landscape for protein folding, misfolding, and aggregation. While, intramolecular contacts may lead protein toward native state. Intermolecular contacts at high protein concentration may causes aggregation (adapted from Singh [29]).

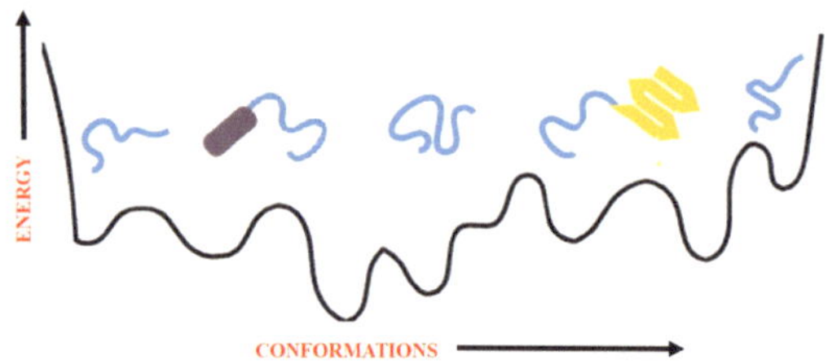

Figure 4.
A representation of the free energy landscape of IDPs. This shows the high-dimensional landscape with multiple low-energy state.

exist in a high-dimensional energy landscape with many low-energy states, as shown in **Figure 4**. The energy landscape of an intrinsically disordered protein is influenced by multiple factors, including interactions with other proteins, small molecules, the environmental condition, and the amino acid sequence of the protein itself. Understanding the energy landscape of intrinsically disordered proteins is essential for understanding their functions and how they interact with other molecules in biological systems [83].

4.1 Intrinsically disordered proteins

In the last couple of decades, a different class of inherently unstructured proteins has been discovered that exhibit substantial evidence for the dynamic nature of proteins [84]. These proteins are engaged in a wide range of cellular processes but lack a single well-defined three-dimensional structure under physiological conditions [85–89]. These proteins are known as "intrinsically disordered proteins" [90]. The term "intrinsically" denotes sequence-dependent qualities, and the term "disordered" is used to designate unstructured regions and covers a wide range of conditions [3, 85, 91, 92]. The intrinsically disordered proteins are characterized by a dynamic ensemble of rapidly interconverting conformations. These proteins are categorized into two groups: (i) intrinsically disordered proteins (IDPs), which have completely disordered sequences and no tertiary structures, and (ii) intrinsically disordered protein regions (IDPRs), which are polypeptide segments without secondary or tertiary structure that are connected to areas with well-defined secondary structures [93]. Thus, according to Wright and Dyson [94], the existence of proteins with intrinsic disorders necessitates a re-evaluation of the protein sequence-structure-function paradigm. Since the amino acid sequence identifies a three-dimensional structure, it should also detect the absence of a 3D structure. Also, if intrinsic disorder underlies certain physiological functions, natural selection must retain the unfolded structure to preserve these functions. Thus, it is necessary to adopt a new paradigm for protein structure-function, termed as the disorder-function paradigm [95–97], to rationalize these possibilities refer to **Figure 5**. IDPs play important roles in various cellular processes, and their importance are widely recognized. The functions of IDPs are given in **Figure 6**.

5. Mechanism of aggregation

Intramolecular interaction is responsible for the folding of protein in the native state, whereas intermolecular interactions between amino acids of different chains may lead to aggregates. Thus, the concentration of protein in the cell plays a vital role in

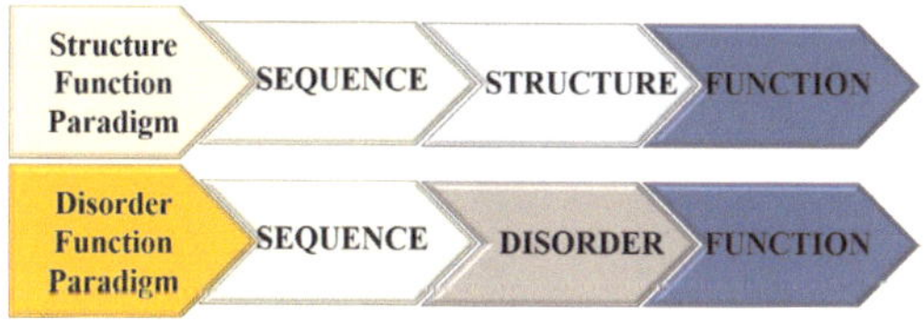

Figure 5.
Sequence to function relationship. Structure-function paradigm and Disorder-function paradigm.

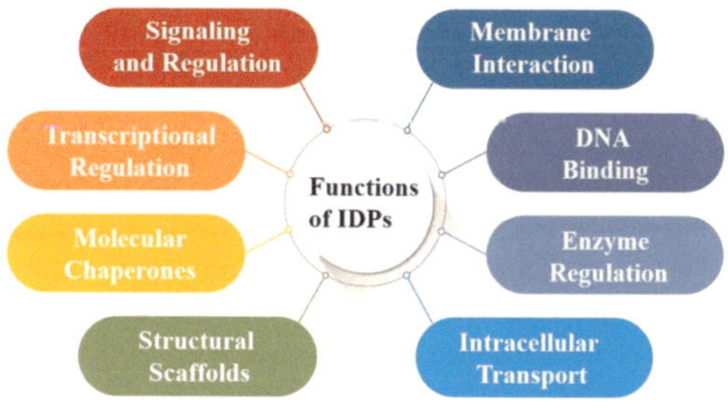

Figure 6.
A schematic representation of the functions of intrinsically disordered proteins.

aggregation. The term critical concentration is introduced as the concentration at which the stability of both aggregate and the native protein becomes equal [98]. The aggregate is only formed when the concentration of protein exceeds the critical value. Several studies consider the misfolded or partially folded segment as the monomer [43, 99, 100]. Factors such as intermolecular interaction [101, 102], increase in β-sheet propensity [103, 104] and the negative consequences of the environment [105, 106] allow the formation of dimer or oligomer from the monomer, which subsequently polymerizes and eventually form the higher order aggregates [107]. Often, these aggregates possess well-defined crystalline structures that are the combination of several β-sheets, known as amyloid fibrils. However, the actual mechanism that defines the aggregation process is not yet clear, but the nucleation growth mechanism is widely accepted by most of the theoretical and experimental studies [43, 99, 100, 107–109].

The nucleation growth mechanism is mainly understood through the following three processes (refer to **Figure 7**).

i. *Nucleation and fragmentation processes*: This is the monomer addition step, where a critical size of the nucleus is formed spontaneously, and this step also determines the reaction order of aggregation due to the slow step. At initial step of this nucleation, the addition of monomer is energetically unfavorable, which implies that all the aggregates having less than their critical size are dissociated/disassembled. Aggregates that are larger than their critical size are energetically favorable and are able to grow effectively. These two processes are associated with the energy barrier. Once the barrier has been overcome as the aggregate size increases above the critical value, the elongation step starts.

ii. *Elongation and dissociation processes*: The size of aggregate can increase and decrease by the addition or removable of single monomer and this step is associated with the change in the number of aggregates, that is, fibrils.

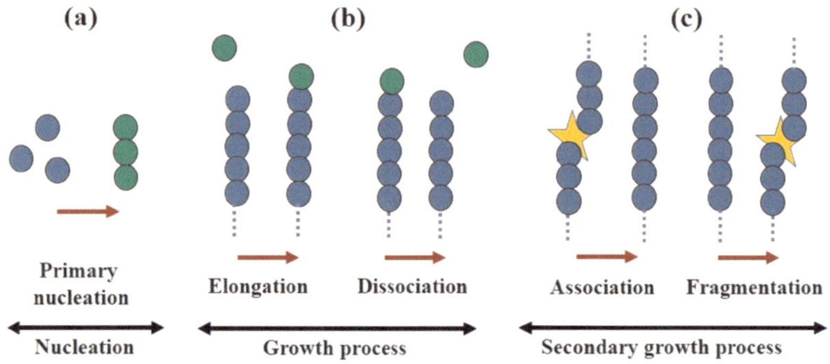

Figure 7.
A schematic diagram of the mechanisms of nucleated polymerization. These three principal classes of elementary mechanisms are defined as (a) primary nucleation processes, (b) growth processes, and (c) secondary growth processes.

iii. *Fragmentation and annealing processes*: Here, the aggregates/fibrils may shrink their size by breaking into smaller filaments or increase their size by the end-to-end association of fibrils.

6. Neurodegenerative disorders

The aggregation prone proteins are mainly natively unfolded or intrinsically disordered proteins that do not exhibit any similarities in sequence, structure, size or function [85, 110]. The misfolding propensity varies from protein to protein depending on the physico-chemical properties of the sequence like hydrophobicity, secondary structure propensity and mean net charge [32, 111]. These proteins have exposed hydrophobic regions that were deeply buried in the folded state and then stabilize their structures by various non-covalent forces like hydrogen bonds, hydrophobic and van der Waals interactions [28, 77–79]. The hydrophobic forces that acts between different protein molecules are the major driving forces for the formation of aggregates. The aggregates are generally amorphous and consist of disordered assemblies of the misfolded proteins. However, they are also found in highly ordered self-associated species of peptides which is known as amyloid fibrils [112–114]. Amyloid fibrils having high Young's modulus and tensile strength [115] consist of β-sheets with a hydrogen-bonded network of cross β-sheet structure in the form of flat ribbons [32, 116–118]; hence, they are highly stable and resilient to degradation [115]. The structure of such aggregates was first given by the biophysicist William Astbury in 1935 [119]. *In vivo*, the amyloids are found in unbranched form with elongated morphology ($\sim 100 - 200$ Å in length) which is rich in β-sheet [120]. The specific architecture of these aggregates is not encoded by their amino acid sequence [36, 121]. Depending on the association mechanism, the aggregates may also exist in other forms like oligomers (small globular aggregates considered as primary toxic species), protofibrils (thin filamentous unit having a high percentage of β-sheet), superstructure (cluster of amyloids) and spherulite (spherical superstructure) [122–124]. The extracellular and/or intracellular deposition of these aggregates in the nervous system causes several age-dependent neurodegenerative disorders [37, 38]. These disorders display several typical features such as neuronal loss, synaptic dysfunction, brain damage, and neuroinflammation which may cause cell death [31, 32].

Three hypotheses have been proposed to understand the protein aggregation with neurodegeneration:

i. *Loss-of-function*: According to this hypothesis, proteins lose their normal activity due to misfolding, which results in protein deficiency diseases. Most disorders such as AD, PD, ALS, and HD belong to this hypothesis and are typically inherited [22, 125, 126].

ii. *Gain-of-function*: On the basis of *in vitro* observations, this hypothesis states that proteins gain neurotoxic function during aggregation. It is the most acceptable hypothesis [127–129].

iii. *Brain inflammation*: This suggests that neurodegeneration is caused by chronic inflammatory reactions in the brain due to the deposition of aggregates [130, 131].

The elimination of the aberrant/misfolded proteins may lead to the loss-of-function pathogenesis, while their extracellular/intracellular accumulation in the brain promotes gain-of-function pathogenesis. However, some disorders show both pathogenic mechanisms. The distribution and composition of protein aggregates are different in each neurodegenerative disease. In AD, plaques [132] of amyloid-β protein are deposited in the extracellular region while, neurofibrillary tangles [133] of tau protein are found in intracellular region of the brain [134, 135]. PD is the second most commonly occurring neurodegenerative disease whose neuropathologic feature consists of Lewy bodies that are composed of α-synuclein [136]. ALS is caused by the aggregation of superoxide dismutase and axons of motor neurons [137]. These diseases are the major threat to human health with the increase in age. Protein aggregation diseases and related misfolded/aggregation pron proteins are given in **Table 1**.

6.1 Alzheimer's disease

Alzheimer's disease (AD) is the most common neurodegenerative disorder, accounting for the majority of cases worldwide and it is characterized by progressive cognitive decline and memory loss. It represents a significant public health challenge globally, affecting millions of individuals. It primarily affects older adults, although early-onset cases also exist. The hallmark pathological features of AD include the accumulation of amyloid-beta (Aβ) plaques outside neurons and neurofibrillary tangles (NFTs) composed of hyperphosphorylated tau protein inside neurons [138–140]. These abnormalities disrupt neuronal communication and contribute to synaptic dysfunction and neurodegeneration. Neuroinflammation, oxidative stress, and mitochondrial dysfunction further exacerbate the disease progression, leading to widespread neuronal loss, particularly in areas of the brain associated with memory and cognitive function [141]. Several risk factors contribute to the development of AD, including age, genetics (e.g., mutations in the amyloid-beta precursor protein (APP), PSEN1, and PSEN2 genes), family history, and lifestyle factors such as cardiovascular health, diet, and physical activity. Apolipoprotein E (APOE) genotype, particularly the $\varepsilon 4$ allele, is strongly associated with increased risk and earlier onset of AD [142–144].

Diagnosing AD typically involves a combination of clinical evaluation, cognitive assessments, neuroimaging (e.g., magnetic resonance imaging (MRI), PET scans), and

S. no.	Diseases	Aggregating protein	Number of residues	Native structure of protein
Neurodegenerative diseases				
1.	Alzheimer's	Amyloid-β	40 or 42	Natively unfolded
2.	Parkinson's	α-Synuclein	140	Natively unfolded
3.	Amyotrophic lateral sclerosis	Superodide dismutase 1	153	All-β
4.	Huntington's	Polyglutamine	47	Natively unfolded
5.	Prion	Prion	230	Natively unfolded and α-helical
6.	Tauopathies	Tau	441	Natively unfolded
7.	Frontotemporal lobar degeneration	TPD43 and ubiquitin	414 and 76	α+β
Peripheral diseases				
8.	Type 2 diabetes	Amylin (IAPP)	37	Natively unfolded
9.	Systemic amyloidosis	Lysozyme	164	α+β
10.	Hemodialysis-related disorder	β2-microglobulin	99	All-β

Table 1.
Protein aggregation diseases.

biomarker analysis (e.g., Aβ42, tau protein in cerebrospinal fluid). Advances in neuroimaging techniques and biomarker research hold promise for early and accurate diagnosis, facilitating timely intervention and personalized treatment strategies. Current treatment approaches for AD focus on symptomatic management and disease modification. Cholinesterase inhibitors (e.g., donepezil, rivastigmine) and N-methyl-D-aspartate (NMDA) receptor antagonists (e.g., memantine) are commonly used to alleviate cognitive symptoms [145–147]. Emerging therapies, however, are focusing on addressing the underlying causes of Alzheimer's disease, such as amyloid-beta (Aβ) and tau protein abnormalities. Clinical trials are underway to evaluate the efficacy of these novel therapies in slowing disease progression and improving cognitive function.

Future research efforts are aimed at unraveling the complex mechanisms underlying AD pathogenesis, identifying novel biomarkers for early diagnosis, and developing targeted therapies. Advancements in genetics, neuroscience, and neuroimaging hold promise for personalized medicine approaches tailored to individual AD profiles. Multidisciplinary collaborations and large-scale initiatives are essential to accelerate progress toward effective prevention and treatment strategies for Alzheimer's disease. Recent advancements in research have shed light on potential biomarkers and therapeutic targets, offering hope for improved management and treatment of this devastating condition.

6.2 Parkinson's disease

Parkinson's disease (PD) is a complex neurodegenerative disorder characterized by progressive loss of dopaminergic neurons in the substantia nigra region of the brain.

This leads to a variety of motor and non-motor symptoms that significantly impact patients' quality of life. The hallmark pathological feature of Parkinson's disease is the presence of Lewy bodies, which are abnormal aggregates of alpha-synuclein protein found within neurons [148, 149]. These Lewy bodies contribute to the degeneration of dopaminergic neurons in the substantia nigra pars compacta, resulting in decreased dopamine levels in the basal ganglia. Dopamine is crucial for regulating motor function, and its deficiency leads to the characteristic motor symptoms of PD, such as bradykinesia (slowness of movement), resting tremor, rigidity, and postural instability [150, 151]. In addition to dopaminergic dysfunction, emerging research suggests that PD involves widespread neuroinflammation, mitochondrial dysfunction, impaired protein degradation pathways, and genetic predisposition factors. These factors contribute to the progressive nature of the disease and the involvement of non-motor symptoms such as cognitive impairment, depression, sleep disturbances, and autonomic dysfunction. Parkinson's disease typically manifests in individuals over the age of 50, although early-onset forms can occur. The cardinal motor symptoms mentioned earlier are often asymmetric in onset and progression. Patients may also experience non-motor symptoms that can precede motor symptoms by several years, complicating early diagnosis.

Diagnosis relies heavily on clinical evaluation, including history-taking and neurological examination, although imaging studies such as dopamine transporter (DAT) scans can provide supportive evidence [152, 153]. The diagnosis of Parkinson's disease is primarily clinical, based on the presence of characteristic motor symptoms and the exclusion of other potential causes. Diagnostic criteria, such as those established by the Movement Disorder Society (MDS), emphasize the importance of assessing both motor and non-motor symptoms to accurately diagnose and stage the disease. Rating scales like the unified Parkinson's disease rating scale (UPDRS) are commonly used to monitor disease progression and assess treatment response [154, 155]. Current treatment strategies for Parkinson's disease aim to alleviate symptoms, enhance quality of life, and potentially modify disease progression. Pharmacological interventions primarily focus on replenishing dopamine levels in the brain through the use of dopamine agonists (e.g., pramipexole and ropinirole), levodopa (converted to dopamine in the brain), and monoamine oxidase-B (MAO-B) inhibitors (e.g., rasagiline and selegiline) [156]. Non-pharmacological approaches, such as physical therapy, speech therapy, and occupational therapy, play crucial roles in managing motor symptoms and improving functional abilities [157]. Surgical options like deep brain stimulation (DBS) are considered for patients with advanced disease who are experiencing motor fluctuations and medication-resistant symptoms [158, 159].

Ongoing research in Parkinson's disease focuses on understanding the mechanisms underlying neurodegeneration, identifying biomarkers for early diagnosis, developing disease-modifying therapies, and exploring non-dopaminergic treatment targets. These efforts aim to improve outcomes, slow disease progression and ultimately find a cure for this debilitating condition. Advances in our understanding of its pathophysiology and treatment approaches continue to evolve, offering hope for better management and, ultimately, a cure for this challenging disease.

6.3 Other NDDs

Neurodegenerative diseases constitute a diverse group of disorders characterized by progressive degeneration of the structure and function of the nervous system. While Alzheimer's disease and Parkinson's disease are well-known, several other conditions also significantly impact neurological health. This note explores some of these lesser-discussed but equally impactful neurodegenerative diseases.

Amyotrophic lateral sclerosis (*ALS*): ALS, also known as Lou Gehrig's disease, affects the motor neurons responsible for voluntary muscle control. It leads to progressive muscle weakness, paralysis, and eventual respiratory failure. The exact cause is often unclear, with both genetic and environmental factors implicated. Research suggests the involvement of protein aggregates, like TDP-43 and SOD1, disrupt cellular functions and lead to neuronal death [160, 161].

Huntington's disease (*HD*): HD is a genetic disorder caused by a mutation in the HTT gene, leading to the production of a toxic form of the huntingtin protein. This results in a gradual deterioration of mental abilities and physical control, including involuntary movements (chorea). HD typically manifests in mid-adulthood, and its progression is relentless, leading to severe disability and, eventually death. Current research focuses on gene silencing therapies and understanding the protein's role in cellular dysfunction [162–165].

Prion diseases: Prion diseases are caused by abnormal, infectious proteins (prions) that induce normal proteins to misfold and accumulate in the brain. Conditions like Creutzfeldt-Jakob disease (CJD) and variant CJD (vCJD) result in rapid neurological deterioration, dementia, and ultimately death. These diseases can be sporadic, inherited, or acquired through exposure to infected tissue, and no effective treatments currently exist [166–168].

Multiple system atrophy (*MSA*): MSA is characterized by the degeneration of multiple areas of the brain, including the basal ganglia, cerebellum, and autonomic nervous system. It presents with symptoms of Parkinsonism, cerebellar ataxia, and autonomic dysfunction, such as orthostatic hypotension and urinary incontinence. The cause remains unclear, though the aggregation of alpha-synuclein protein is implicated in neuronal death and dysfunction [169, 170].

Frontotemporal dementia (*FTD*): FTD encompasses a group of disorders affecting the frontal and temporal lobes of the brain, leading to progressive changes in behavior, personality, and language abilities. Unlike Alzheimer's disease, which primarily affects memory, FTD primarily impacts social conduct and decision-making abilities. It is associated with abnormal protein accumulations, such as tau and TDP-43, contributing to neuronal loss and cognitive decline [171, 172].

Understanding the diverse nature of neurodegenerative diseases beyond Alzheimer's and Parkinson's is crucial for advancing diagnostic techniques and therapeutic strategies. Each of these conditions presents unique challenges, from genetic predisposition to protein aggregation and neuronal dysfunction. Ongoing research aims to uncover underlying mechanisms, develop targeted therapies, and improve the quality of life for affected individuals.

7. Conclusions

Neurodegenerative diseases, such as Alzheimer's, Parkinson's, and Huntington's diseases, are marked by the progressive loss of neuronal function and structure. Central to their pathogenesis is the disruption of protein turnover and the consequent accumulation of misfolded proteins. Protein quality control, protein turnover, and molecular chaperones play a pivotal role in maintaining protein homeostasis by ensuring proper protein folding and the degradation of misfolded proteins. Failures within this network lead to the buildup of toxic protein aggregates, which is a hallmark of neurodegenerative diseases. From a thermodynamic perspective, proteins fold into their native, functional states by traversing a complex free energy landscape, where the native state is typically the global minimum. In neurodegenerative diseases, this landscape is altered, causing proteins to become trapped in local minima, which correspond to stable yet dysfunctional misfolded states or aggregates. These misfolded proteins often form insoluble fibrillar aggregates, such as amyloid-beta plaques in Alzheimer's disease or alpha-synuclein in Parkinson's disease, which are resistant to proteolytic degradation and toxic to cells. Genetic mutations can further destabilize protein structures, increasing their propensity to misfold and aggregate. For instance, mutations in the APP (amyloid-beta precursor protein) gene associated with Alzheimer's disease result in abnormal processing of amyloid precursor protein, leading to amyloid-beta accumulation. Additionally, environmental factors such as oxidative stress, pH, temperature, and pressure exacerbate protein misfolding by inducing structural damage or modifying the energy landscape, overwhelming the cell's proteostasis capacity.

The toxic species formed by misfolded proteins and their aggregates can impair numerous cellular functions. They disrupt membrane integrity, impair mitochondrial function, interfere with synaptic signaling, and induce inflammatory responses. These disruptions lead to neuronal dysfunction and eventual cell death. Understanding the intricate interplay between protein turnover, free energy landscapes, and the resulting cellular mechanisms in neurodegenerative diseases is crucial for developing therapeutic strategies. Potential interventions aim to enhance proteostasis, stabilize protein conformations, or facilitate the clearance of toxic aggregates, offering hope for mitigating the progression of these debilitating diseases.

Since, the animal models have their own limitations that may be filled up by understanding the theoretical aspects of protein misfolding and aggregation, which provide valuable insights into the pathogenesis of these disorders and informs the development of potential therapeutic strategies. The massive development of digital data and computational and mathematical methods allows us to build an adequate model of biological systems and related diseases to gain insight into neurodegeneration. These models may assist in the discovery of novel biomarkers in neurodegeneration that may provide an earlier diagnosis before the development of neurological symptoms. As research continues to unravel the molecular mechanisms underlying protein aggregation, new opportunities for intervention may emerge, offering hope for patients suffering from these debilitating conditions.

Acknowledgements

Vishal Singh acknowledges the Delhi School of Public Health, Institution of Eminence, University of Delhi, for providing the lab space and other facilities for work.

Conflict of interest

The authors declare no conflict of interest.

Abbreviations

PQC	protein quality control
HSP	Heat SHOCK protein
IDP	intrinsically disordered protein
FEL	free energy landscape
NDDs	neurodegenerative disorders
AD	Alzheimer's disease
PD	Parkinson's disease
ALS	amyotrophic lateral sclerosis
HD	Huntington's disease
CJD	Creutzfeldt-Jakob disease
MSA	multiple system strophy
FTD	frontotemporal dementia
$A\beta$	amyloid-beta
NFT	neurofibrillary tangles
MDS	movement disorder society
DBS	deep brain stimulation

Author details

Vishal Singh[1]* and Priya Dey[2]

1 Discipline in Chemistry, School of Sciences, Indira Gandhi National Open University, Maidan Garhi, New Delhi, India

2 Deenbandhu Chhotu Ram University of Science and Technology, Sonipat, Haryana, India

*Address all correspondence to: vishalsingh@ignou.ac.in

References

[1] Whitford D. Proteins: Structure and Function. England: John Wiley & Sons; 2013

[2] Petsko GA, Ringe D. Protein Structure and Function. London: New Science Press; 2004

[3] Dyson HJ, Wright PE. Intrinsically unstructured proteins and their functions. Nature Reviews. Molecular Cell Biology. 2005;**6**:197-208

[4] Finkelstein AV, Ptitsyn O. Protein Physics: A Course of Lectures. London: Academic Press; 2016

[5] Prowle JR, Echeverri JE, Ligabo EV, Ronco C, Bellomo R. Fluid balance and acute kidney injury. Nature Reviews. Nephrology. 2010;**6**:107-115

[6] Pace CN. Contribution of the hydrophobic effect to globular protein stability. Journal of Molecular Biology. 1992;**226**:29-35

[7] Lins L, Brasseur R. The hydrophobic effect in protein folding. The FASEB Journal. 1995;**9**:535-540

[8] Kronberg B. The hydrophobic effect. Current Opinion in Colloid & Interface Science. 2016;**22**:14-22

[9] Levinthal C. Are there pathways for protein folding? Journal de Chimie Physique. 1968;**65**:44-45

[10] Zwanzig R, Szabo A, Bagchi B. Levinthal's paradox. Proceedings of the National Academy of Sciences of the United States of America. 1992;**89**:20-22

[11] Singh V, Biswas P. Estimating the mean first passage time of protein misfolding. Physical Chemistry Chemical Physics. 2018;**20**:5692-5698

[12] Singh V, Biswas P. Predicting protein shelf lives from mean first passage times. Chemical Physics Letters. 2022;**792**: 139426

[13] Eaton WA, Munoz V, Thompson PA, Henry ER, Hofrichter J. Kinetics and dynamics of loops, -helices, -hairpins, and fast-folding proteins. Accounts of Chemical Research. 1998;**31**:745-754

[14] Eaton WA, Muñoz V, Hagen SJ, Jas GS, Lapidus LJ, Henry ER, et al. Fast kinetics and mechanisms in protein folding. Annual Review of Biophysics and Biomolecular Structure. 2000;**29**: 327-359

[15] Mori T, Saito S. Molecular mechanism behind the fast folding/unfolding transitions of villin headpiece subdomain: Hierarchy and heterogeneity. The Journal of Physical Chemistry. B. 2016;**120**:11683-11691

[16] Prigozhin M, Gruebele M. Microsecond folding experiments and simulations: A match is made. Physical Chemistry Chemical Physics. 2013;**15**: 3372-3388

[17] Dill KA, Chan HS. From Levinthal to pathways to funnels. Nature Structural Biology. 1997;**4**:10-19

[18] Onuchic JN, Wolynes PG. Theory of protein folding. Current Opinion in Structural Biology. 2004;**14**:70-75

[19] Frauenfelder H, Leeson DT. The energy landscape in non-biological and biological molecules. Nature Structural Biology. 1998;**5**:757-759

[20] Dill KA, MacCallum JL. The protein-folding problem, 50 years on. Science. 2012;**338**:1042-1046

[21] Dill KA, Ozkan SB, Shell MS, Weikl TR. The protein folding problem. Annual Review of Biophysics. 2008;**37**:289-316

[22] Gregersen N, Bross P, Vang S, Christensen JH. Protein misfolding and human disease. Annual Review of Genomics and Human Genetics. 2006;**7**: 103-124

[23] Dill KA. Dominant forces in protein folding. Biochemistry. 1990;**29**:7133-7155

[24] Newberry RW, Raines RT. Secondary forces in protein folding. ACS Chemical Biology. 2019;**14**:1677-1686

[25] Amm I, Sommer T, Wolf DH. Protein quality control and elimination of protein waste: The role of the ubiquitin–proteasome system. Biochimica et Biophysica Acta. 2014; **1843**:182-196

[26] Hartl FU, Hayer-Hartl M. Molecular chaperones in the cytosol: From nascent chain to folded protein. Science. 2002; **295**:1852-1858

[27] Cho Y, Zhang X, Pobre KFR, Liu Y, Powers DL, Kelly JW, et al. Individual and collective contributions of chaperoning and degradation to protein homeostasis in *E. coli*. Cell Reports. 2015; **11**:321-333

[28] Ellis RJ, Pinheiro TJ. Danger—misfolding proteins. Nature. 2002;**416**: 483-484

[29] Singh V. Stochastic dynamics of protein misfolding and aggregation [thesis]. Delhi: University of Delhi; 2020. p. 16

[30] Kelly JW. Alternative conformations of amyloidogenic proteins govern their behavior. Current Opinion in Structural Biology. 1996;**6**:11-17

[31] Vaquer-Alicea J, Diamond MI. Propagation of protein aggregation in neurodegenerative diseases. Annual Review of Biochemistry. 2019;**88**: 785-810

[32] Chiti F, Dobson CM. Protein misfolding, functional amyloid, and human disease. Annual Review of Biochemistry. 2006;**75**:333-366

[33] Holmes BB, Furman JL, Mahan TE, Yamasaki TR, Mirbaha H, Eades WC, et al. Proteopathic tau seeding predicts tauopathy in vivo. Proceedings. National Academy of Sciences. United States of America. 2014;**111**:E4376-E4385

[34] Enam C, Geffen Y, Ravid T, Gardner RG. Protein quality control degradation in the nucleus. Annual Review of Biochemistry. 2018;**87**:725-749

[35] Pedersen JT, Heegaard NH. Analysis of protein aggregation in neurodegenerative disease. Analytical Chemistry. 2013;**85**:4215-4227

[36] Dobson CM. Protein folding and misfolding. Nature. 2003;**426**:884-890

[37] Ross CA, Poirier MA. Protein aggregation and neurodegenerative disease. Nature Medicine. 2004;**10**: S10-S17

[38] Soto C. Unfolding the role of protein misfolding in neurodegenerative diseases. Nature Reviews. Neuroscience. 2003;**4**:49-60

[39] Eisenberg D, Nelson R, Sawaya MR, Balbirnie M, Sambashivan S, Ivanova MI, et al. The structural biology of protein aggregation diseases: Fundamental questions and some answers. Accounts of Chemical Research. 2006;**39**:568-575

[40] Ellis RJ. Macromolecular crowding: An important but neglected aspect of the intracellular environment. Current

Opinion in Structural Biology. 2001;**11**: 114-119

[41] Chi EY, Krishnan S, Randolph TW, Carpenter JF. Physical stability of proteins in aqueous solution: Mechanism and driving forces in nonnative protein aggregation. Pharmaceutical Research. 2003;**20**:1325-1336

[42] Wang W, Nema S, Teagarden D. Protein aggregation-pathways and influencing factors. International Journal of Pharmaceutics. 2010;**390**:89-99

[43] Biswas P. Theoretical and computational advances in protein misfolding. In: Advances in Protein Chemistry and Structural Biology. Vol. 118. London: Elsevier; 2020. pp. 1-31

[44] Chiti F, Calamai M, Taddei N, Stefani M, Ramponi G, Dobson CM. Studies of the aggregation of mutant proteins in vitro provide insights into the genetics of amyloid diseases. Proceedings. National Academy of Sciences. United States of America. 2002;**99**:16419-16426

[45] Hartl FU, Hayer-Hartl M. Converging concepts of protein folding in vitro and in vivo. Nature Structural & Molecular Biology. 2009;**16**:574-581

[46] Hartl FU. Molecular chaperones in cellular protein folding. Nature. 1996; **381**:571-580

[47] Garrido C, Gurbuxani S, Ravagnan L, Kroemer G. Heat shock proteins: Endogenous modulators of apoptotic cell death. Biochemical and Biophysical Research Communications. 2001;**286**: 433-442

[48] Ciechanover A, Kwon YT. Protein quality control by molecular chaperones in neurodegeneration. Frontiers in Neuroscience. 2017;**11**:185

[49] Ranford JC, Coates AR, Henderson B. Chaperonins are cell-signalling proteins: The unfolding biology of molecular chaperones. Expert Reviews in Molecular Medicine. 2000;**2**:1-17

[50] Tutar L, Tutar Y. Heat shock proteins; an overview. Current Pharmaceutical Biotechnology. 2010;**11**: 216-222

[51] DeSantis ME, Leung EH, Sweeny EA, Jackrel ME, Cushman-Nick M, Neuhaus-Follini A, et al. Operational plasticity enables hsp104 to disaggregate diverse amyloid and nonamyloid clients. Cell. 2012;**151**:778-793

[52] Bianco CL, Shorter J, Régulier E, Lashuel H, Iwatsubo T, Lindquist S, et al. Hsp104 antagonizes α-synuclein aggregation and reduces dopaminergic degeneration in a rat model of Parkinson disease. The Journal of Clinical Investigation. 2008;**118**:3087-3097

[53] Kaestle M, Grune T. Interactions of the proteasomal system with chaperones: Protein triage and protein quality control. Progress in Molecular Biology and Translational Science. 2012;**109**: 113-160

[54] Hartl FU, Bracher A, Hayer-Hartl M. Molecular chaperones in protein folding and proteostasis. Nature. 2011;**475**: 324-332

[55] Toyama BH, Hetzer MW. Protein homeostasis: Live long, won't prosper. Nature Reviews. Molecular Cell Biology. 2013;**14**:55-61

[56] Rothman S. How is the balance between protein synthesis and degradation achieved? Theoretical Biology and Medical Modelling. 2010;**7**:25

[57] Goldberg AL. Protein degradation and protection against misfolded or

damaged proteins. Nature. 2003;**426**: 895-899

[58] Glickman MH, Ciechanover A. The ubiquitin-proteasome proteolytic pathway: Destruction for the sake of construction. Physiological Reviews. 2002;**82**:373-428

[59] Belle A, Tanay A, Bitincka L, Shamir R, O'Shea EK. Quantification of protein half-lives in the budding yeast proteome. Proceedings. National Academy of Sciences. United States of America. 2006;**103**:13004-13009

[60] Yen H-CS, Xu Q, Chou DM, Zhao Z, Elledge SJ. Global protein stability profiling in mammalian cells. Science. 2008;**322**:918-923

[61] Cambridge SB, Gnad F, Nguyen C, Bermejo JL, KruÌˆger M, Mann M. Systems-wide proteomic analysis in mammalian cells reveals conserved, functional protein turnover. Journal of Proteome Research. 2011;**10**: 5275-5284

[62] Karplus M. The Levinthal paradox: Yesterday and today. Folding & Design. 1997;**2**:S69-S75

[63] Wolynes PG, Onuchic JN, Thirumalai D. Navigating the folding routes. Science. 1995;**267**:1619-1620

[64] Frauenfelder H, Sligar SG, Wolynes PG. The energy landscapes and motions of proteins. Science. 1991;**254**:1598-1603

[65] Bryngelson JD, Wolynes PG. Spin glasses and the statistical mechanics of protein folding. Proceedings. National Academy of Sciences. United States of America. 1987;**84**:7524-7528

[66] Dill KA. Polymer principles and protein folding. Protein Science. 1999;**8**: 1166-1180

[67] Dill KA, Alonso DO, Hutchinson K. Thermal stabilities of globular proteins. Biochemistry. 1989;**28**:5439-5449

[68] Leopold PE, Montal M, Onuchic JN. Protein folding funnels: A kinetic approach to the sequence-structure relationship. Proceedings. National Academy of Sciences. United States of America. 1992;**89**:8721-8725

[69] Onuchic JN, Luthey-Schulten Z, Wolynes PG. Theory of protein folding: The energy landscape perspective. Annual Review of Physical Chemistry. 1997;**48**:545-600

[70] Ferreiro DU, Hegler JA, Komives EA, Wolynes PG. Localizing frustration in native proteins and protein assemblies. Proceedings. National Academy of Sciences. United States of America. 2007;**104**:19819-19824

[71] Vendruscolo M, Paci E, Karplus M, Dobson CM. Structures and relative free energies of partially folded states of proteins. Proceedings. National Academy of Sciences. United States of America. 2003;**100**:14817-14821

[72] Brockwell DJ, Radford SE. Intermediates: Ubiquitous species on folding energy landscapes? Current Opinion in Structural Biology. 2007;**17**: 30-37

[73] Thirumalai D, Woodson S. Kinetics of folding of proteins and RNA. Accounts of Chemical Research. 1996;**29**: 433-439

[74] Singh V, Biswas P. A generalized Langevin equation approach for barrier crossing dynamics in conformational transitions of proteins. Journal of Statistical Mechanics. 2021; **2021**:063502

[75] Frydman J. Folding of newly translated proteins in vivo: The role of molecular chaperones. Annual Review of Biochemistry. 2001;**70**:603-647

[76] Jahn TR, Radford SE. Folding versus aggregation: Polypeptide conformations on competing pathways. Archives of Biochemistry and Biophysics. 2008;**469**: 100-117

[77] Meric G, Robinson AS, Roberts CJ. Driving forces for nonnative protein aggregation and approaches to predict aggregation-prone regions. Annual Review of Chemical and Biomolecular Engineering. 2017;**8**:139-159

[78] Thirumalai D, Reddy G, Straub JE. Role of water in protein aggregation and amyloid polymorphism. Accounts of Chemical Research. 2012;**45**:83-92

[79] Chong S-H, Ham S. Distinct role of hydration water in protein misfolding and aggregation revealed by fluctuating thermodynamics analysis. Accounts of Chemical Research. 2015;**48**:956-965

[80] Clark PL. Protein folding in the cell: Reshaping the folding funnel. Trends in Biochemical Sciences. 2004;**29**:527-534

[81] Jahn TR, Radford SE. The Yin and Yang of protein folding. The FEBS Journal. 2005;**272**:5962-5970

[82] Balchin D, Hayer-Hartl M, Hartl FU. In vivo aspects of protein folding and quality control. Science. 2016;**353**: aac4354

[83] Singh V, Biswas P. Conformational transitions of amyloid-β: A Langevin and generalized Langevin dynamics simulation study. ACS Omega. 2021;**6**: 13611-13619

[84] Dunker AK, Silman I, Uversky VN, Sussman JL. Function and structure of inherently disordered proteins. Current Opinion in Structural Biology. 2008;**18**: 756-764

[85] Van Der Lee R, Buljan M, Lang B, Weatheritt RJ, Daughdrill GW, Dunker AK, et al. Classification of intrinsically disordered regions and proteins. Chemical Reviews. 2014;**114**:6589-6631

[86] Dunker AK, Brown CJ, Lawson JD, Iakoucheva LM, Obradović Z. Intrinsic disorder and protein function. Biochemistry. 2002;**41**:6573-6582

[87] Tompa P. The interplay between structure and function in intrinsically unstructured proteins. FEBS Letters. 2005;**579**:3346-3354

[88] Dunker AK, Oldfield CJ, Meng J, Romero P, Yang JY, Chen JW, et al. The unfoldomics decade: An update on intrinsically disordered proteins. BMC Genomics. 2008;**9**:1-26

[89] Dunker AK, Lawson JD, Brown CJ, Williams RM, Romero P, Oh JS, et al. Intrinsically disordered protein. Journal of Molecular Graphics & Modelling. 2001;**19**:26-59

[90] Dunker AK, Babu MM, Barbar E, Blackledge M, Bondos SE, Dosztányi Z, et al. What's in a name? Why these proteins are intrinsically disordered: Why these proteins are intrinsically disordered. Intrinsically Disordered Proteins. 2013;**1**:e24157

[91] Coskuner-Weber O, Mirzanli O, Uversky VN. Intrinsically disordered proteins and proteins with intrinsically disordered regions in neurodegenerative diseases. Biophysical Reviews. 2022;**14**: 679-707

[92] Fink AL. Natively unfolded proteins. Current Opinion in Structural Biology. 2005;**15**:35-41

[93] Uversky VN, Oldfield CJ, Dunker AK. Intrinsically disordered proteins in human diseases: Introducing the D2 concept. Annual Review of Biophysics. 2008;**37**:215-246

[94] Wright PE, Dyson HJ. Intrinsically unstructured proteins: Re-assessing the protein structure-function paradigm. Journal of Molecular Biology. 1999;**293**: 321-331

[95] Zhou J, Oldfield CJ, Yan W, Shen B, Dunker AK. Intrinsically disordered domains: Sequence→disorder→function relationships. Protein Science. 2019;**28**: 1652-1663

[96] Wang W. Recent advances in atomic molecular dynamics simulation of intrinsically disordered proteins. Physical Chemistry Chemical Physics. 2021;**23**:777-784

[97] Uversky VN. Protein intrinsic disorder and structure-function continuum. Progress in Molecular Biology and Translational Science. 2019; **166**:1-17

[98] Baldwin AJ, Knowles TP, Tartaglia GG, Fitzpatrick AW, Devlin GL, Shammas SL, et al. Metastability of native proteins and the phenomenon of amyloid formation. Journal of the American Chemical Society. 2011;**133**: 14160-14163

[99] Knowles TP, Waudby CA, Devlin GL, Cohen SI, Aguzzi A, Vendruscolo M, et al. An analytical solution to the kinetics of breakable filament assembly. Science. 2009;**326**:1533-1537

[100] Morris AM, Watzky MA, Finke RG. Protein aggregation kinetics, mechanism, and curve-fitting: A review of the literature. Biochimica et Biophysica Acta (BBA) - Proteins and Proteomics. 2009;**1794**:375-397

[101] Esfandiary R, Parupudi A, Casas-Finet J, Gadre D, Sathish H. Mechanism of reversible self-association of a monoclonal antibody: Role of electrostatic and hydrophobic interactions. Journal of Pharmaceutical Sciences. 2015;**104**:577-586

[102] Arzensek D, Kuzman D, Podgornik R. Hofmeister effects in monoclonal antibody solution interactions. The Journal of Physical Chemistry. B. 2015; **119**:10375-10389

[103] Krause ME, Martin TT, Laurence JS. Mapping site-specific changes that affect stability of the N-terminal domain of calmodulin. Molecular Pharmaceutics. 2012;**9**:734-743

[104] Bemporad F, De Simone A, Chiti F, Dobson CM. Characterizing intermolecular interactions that initiate native-like protein aggregation. Biophysical Journal. 2012;**102**:2595-2604

[105] Gidalevitz T, Prahlad V, Morimoto RI. The stress of protein misfolding: From single cells to multicellular organisms. Cold Spring Harbor Perspectives in Biology. 2011;**3**:a009704

[106] Stefani M. Protein misfolding and aggregation: New examples in medicine and biology of the dark side of the protein world. Biochimica et Biophysica Acta. 2004;**1739**:5-25

[107] Wang W, Roberts CJ. Protein aggregation–mechanisms, detection, and control. International Journal of Pharmaceutics. 2018;**550**:251-268

[108] Cohen SI, Vendruscolo M, Dobson CM, Knowles TP. From macroscopic measurements to microscopic mechanisms of protein aggregation. Journal of Molecular Biology. 2012;**421**: 160-171

[109] Chatani E, Yamamoto N. Recent progress on understanding the mechanisms of amyloid nucleation. Biophysical Reviews. 2018;**10**:527-534

[110] Soto C, Pritzkow S. Protein misfolding, aggregation, and conformational strains in neurodegenerative diseases. Nature Neuroscience. 2018;**21**:1332-1340

[111] Chiti F, Stefani M, Taddei N, Ramponi G, Dobson CM. Rationalization of the effects of mutations on peptide andprotein aggregation rates. Nature. 2003;**424**:805-808

[112] Serio TR, Cashikar AG, Kowal AS, Sawicki GJ, Moslehi JJ, Serpell L, et al. Nucleated conformational conversion and the replication of conformational information by a prion determinant. Science. 2000;**289**:1317-1321

[113] Knowles TP, Vendruscolo M, Dobson CM. The amyloid state and its association with protein misfolding diseases. Nature Reviews. Molecular Cell Biology. 2014;**15**:384-396

[114] Prusiner SB. Prions. Proceedings of the National Academy of Sciences of the United States of America. 1998;**95**:13363-13383

[115] Knowles TP, Fitzpatrick AW, Meehan S, Mott HR, Vendruscolo M, Dobson CM, et al. Role of intermolecular forces in defining material properties of protein nanofibrils. Science. 2007;**318**: 1900-1903

[116] Hartl FU. Protein misfolding diseases. Annual Review of Biochemistry. 2017;**86**:21-26

[117] Qiang W, Yau W-M, Luo Y, Mattson MP, Tycko R. Antiparallel β-sheet architecture in Iowa-mutant β-amyloid fibrils. Proceedings. National Academy of Sciences. United States of America. 2012;**109**:4443-4448

[118] Jahn TR, Makin OS, Morris KL, Marshall KE, Tian P, Sikorski P, et al. The common architecture of cross-β amyloid. Journal of Molecular Biology. 2010;**395**:717-727

[119] Astbury WT, Dickinson S, Bailey K. The X-ray interpretation of denaturation and the structure of the seed globulins. The Biochemical Journal. 1935;**29**: 2351-2360

[120] Fitzpatrick AW, Debelouchina GT, Bayro MJ, Clare DK, Caporini MA, Bajaj VS, et al. Atomic structure and hierarchical assembly of a cross-β amyloid fibril. Proceedings. National Academy of Sciences. United States of America. 2013;**110**:5468-5473

[121] Dobson CM. Protein misfolding, evolution and disease. Trends in Biochemical Sciences. 1999;**24**:329-332

[122] Vetri V, Foderà V. The route to protein aggregate superstructures: Particulates and amyloid-like spherulites. FEBS Letters. 2015;**589**: 2448-2463

[123] Krebs MR, Domike KR, Donald AM. Protein aggregation: More than just fibrils. Biochemical Society Transactions. 2009;**37**:682-686

[124] Foderà V, Zaccone A, Lattuada M, Donald AM. Electrostatics controls the formation of amyloid superstructures in protein aggregation. Physical Review Letters. 2013;**111**:108105

[125] Cattaneo E, Rigamonti D, Goffredo D, Zuccato C, Squitieri F, Sipione S. Loss of normal huntingtin function: New developments in Huntington's disease research. Trends in Neurosciences. 2001; **24**:182-188

[126] Martins VR, Linden R, Prado MA, Walz R, Sakamoto AC, Izquierdo I, et al. Cellular prion protein: On the road for functions. FEBS Letters. 2002;**512**:25-28

[127] Loo DT, Copani A, Pike CJ, Whittemore ER, Walencewicz AJ, Cotman CW. Apoptosis is induced by beta-amyloid in cultured central nervous system neurons. Proceedings. National Academy of Sciences. United States of America. 1993;**90**:7951-7955

[128] Forloni G, Angeretti N, Chiesa R, Monzani E, Salmona M, Bugiani O, et al. Neurotoxicity of a prion protein fragment. Nature. 1993;**362**:543-546

[129] Lunkes A, Mandel J-L. A cellular model that recapitulates major pathogenic steps of Huntington's disease. Human Molecular Genetics. 1998;7:1 355-1361

[130] Xia M, Hyman BT. Chemokines/ chemokine receptors in the central nervous system and Alzheimer's disease. Journal of Neurovirology. 1999;5:32-41

[131] Wyss-Coray T, Mucke L. Inflammation in neurodegenerative disease—A double-edged sword. Neuron. 2002;**35**:419-432

[132] Glenner GG, Wong CW. Alzheimer's disease: Initial report of the purification and characterization of a novel cerebrovascular amyloid protein. Biochemical and Biophysical Research Communications. 1984;**120**:885-890

[133] Grundke-Iqbal I, Iqbal K, Quinlan M, Tung Y-C, Zaidi MS, Wisniewski HM, et al. A component of Alzheimer paired helical filaments. The Journal of Biological Chemistry. 1986;**261**:6084-6089

[134] Groh N, Bühler A, Huang C, Li KW, van Nierop P, Smit AB, et al. Age-dependent protein aggregation initiates amyloid-β aggregation. Frontiers in Aging Neuroscience. 2017;**9**:138

[135] McKhann GM, Knopman DS, Chertkow H, Hyman BT, Jack CR Jr, Kawas CH, et al. The diagnosis of dementia due to Alzheimer's disease: Recommendations from the National Institute on Aging-Alzheimer's association workgroups on diagnostic guidelines for Alzheimer's disease. Alzheimer's & Dementia. 2011;7:263-269

[136] Spillantini MG, Schmidt ML, Lee VM-Y, Trojanowski JQ, Jakes R, Goedert M. α-Synuclein in Lewy bodies. Nature. 1997;**388**:839-840

[137] Bruijn LI, Houseweart MK, Kato S, Anderson KL, Anderson SD, Ohama E, et al. Aggregation and motor neuron toxicity of an ALS-linked SOD1 mutant independent from wild-type SOD1. Science. 1998;**281**:1851-1854

[138] Knopman DS, Amieva H, Petersen RC, Chételat G, Holtzman DM, Hyman BT, et al. Alzheimer disease. Nature Reviews Disease Primers. 2021;7:33

[139] Serrano-Pozo A, Frosch MP, Masliah E, Hyman BT. Neuropathological alterations in Alzheimer disease. Cold Spring Harbor Perspectives in Medicine. 2011;**1**: a006189

[140] Reitz C, Brayne C, Mayeux R. Epidemiology of Alzheimer disease. Nature Reviews. Neurology. 2011;7: 137-152

[141] Mayeux R, Stern Y. Epidemiology of Alzheimer disease. Cold Spring Harbor Perspectives in Medicine. 2012;**2**: a006239

[142] Tsai M, Tangalos EG, Petersen RC, Smith GE, Schaid DJ, Kokmen E, et al.

Apolipoprotein E: Risk factor for Alzheimer disease. American Journal of Human Genetics. 1994;**54**:643

[143] Verghese PB, Castellano JM, Holtzman DM. Apolipoprotein E in Alzheimer's disease and other neurological disorders. Lancet Neurology. 2011;**10**:241-252

[144] Yamazaki Y, Zhao N, Caulfield TR, Liu C-C, Bu G. Apolipoprotein E and Alzheimer disease: Pathobiology and targeting strategies. Nature Reviews. Neurology. 2019;**15**:501-518

[145] Olivares D, Deshpande VK, Shi Y, Lahiri DK, Greig NH, Rogers JT, et al. N-methyl D-aspartate (NMDA) receptor antagonists and memantine treatment for Alzheimer's disease, vascular dementia and Parkinson's disease. Current Alzheimer Research. 2012;**9**: 746-758

[146] Geerts H, Grossberg GT. Pharmacology of acetylcholinesterase inhibitors and N-methyl-D-aspartate receptors for combination therapy in the treatment of Alzheimer's disease. Journal of Clinical Pharmacology. 2006;**46**: 8S-16S

[147] Finn L. Current medications for the treatment of Alzheimer's disease: Acetylcholinesterase inhibitors and NMDA receptor antagonist. In: Drug Discovery Approaches for the Treatment of Neurodegenerative Disorders. London: Academic Press; 2017. pp. 49-58

[148] Schulz-Schaeffer WJ. The synaptic pathology of α-synuclein aggregation in dementia with Lewy bodies, Parkinson's disease and Parkinson's disease dementia. Acta Neuropathologica. 2010; **120**:131-143

[149] Ingelsson M. Alpha-synuclein oligomers—Neurotoxic molecules in Parkinson's disease and other Lewy body disorders. Frontiers in Neuroscience. 2016;**10**:408

[150] Latif S, Jahangeer M, Razia DM, Ashiq M, Ghaffar A, Akram M, et al. Dopamine in Parkinson's disease. Clinica Chimica Acta. 2021;**522**:114-126

[151] Mishra A, Singh S, Shukla S. Physiological and functional basis of dopamine receptors and their role in neurogenesis: Possible implication for Parkinson's disease. Journal of Experimental Neuroscience. 2018;**12**: 1179069518779829

[152] Porter E, Roussakis A-A, Lao-Kaim NP, Piccini P. Multimodal dopamine transporter (DAT) imaging and magnetic resonance imaging (MRI) to characterise early Parkinson's disease. Parkinsonism & Related Disorders. 2020;**79**:26-33

[153] Brücke T, Brücke C. Dopamine transporter (DAT) imaging in Parkinson's disease and related disorders. Journal of Neural Transmission. 2022; **129**:581-594

[154] Movement Disorder Society Task Force on Rating Scales for Parkinson's Disease. The unified Parkinson's disease rating scale (UPDRS): Status and recommendations. Movement Disorders. 2003;**18**:738-750

[155] Shulman LM, Gruber-Baldini AL, Anderson KE, Fishman PS, Reich SG, Weiner WJ. The clinically important difference on the unified Parkinson's disease rating scale. Archives of Neurology. 2010;**67**:64-70

[156] Perez-Lloret S, Rascol O. Dopamine receptor agonists for the treatment of early or advanced Parkinson's disease. CNS Drugs. 2010;**24**:941-968

[157] Casarotto RA, de Andrade CRF, Tanaka C, Lancman S, Oliver FC. Physical therapy, speech therapy and occupational therapy: Past, present and future. Revista Médica. 2016;**95**:29-34

[158] Machado A, Rezai AR, Kopell BH, Gross RE, Sharan AD, Benabid A-L. Deep brain stimulation for Parkinson's disease: Surgical technique and perioperative management. Journal of Movement Disorders. 2006;**21**:S247-S258

[159] Hickey P, Stacy M. Deep brain stimulation: A paradigm shifting approach to treat Parkinson's disease. Frontiers in Neuroscience. 2016;**10**:173

[160] Baloh RH. TDP-43: The relationship between protein aggregation and neurodegeneration in amyotrophic lateral sclerosis and frontotemporal lobar degeneration. The FEBS Journal. 2011; **278**:3539-3549

[161] Prasad A, Bharathi V, Sivalingam V, Girdhar A, Patel BK. Molecular mechanisms of TDP-43 misfolding and pathology in amyotrophic lateral sclerosis. Frontiers in Molecular Neuroscience. 2019;**12**:25

[162] Stoker TB, Mason SL, Greenland JC, Holden ST, Santini H, Barker RA. Huntington's disease: Diagnosis and management. Practical Neurology. 2022; **22**:32-41

[163] Tabrizi SJ, Schobel S, Gantman EC, Mansbach A, Borowsky B, Konstantinova P, et al. A biological classification of Huntington's disease: The integrated staging system. Lancet Neurology. 2022;**21**:632-644

[164] Tabrizi SJ, Estevez-Fraga C, van Roon-Mom WM, Flower MD, Scahill RI, Wild EJ, et al. Potential disease-modifying therapies for Huntington's disease: Lessons learned and future opportunities. Lancet Neurology. 2022; **21**:645-658

[165] Quarrell O. Huntington's Disease. Oxford: Oxford University Press; 2020

[166] Zhu C, Aguzzi A. Prion protein and prion disease at a glance. Journal of Cell Science. 2021;**134**:jcs245605

[167] Vallabh SM, Minikel EV, Schreiber SL, Lander ES. Towards a treatment for genetic prion disease: Trials and biomarkers. Lancet Neurology. 2020;**19**: 361-368

[168] Appleby BS, Shetty S, Elkasaby M. Genetic aspects of human prion diseases. Frontiers in Neurology. 2022;**13**:1003056

[169] Poewe W, Stankovic I, Halliday G, Meissner WG, Wenning GK, Pellecchia MT, et al. Multiple system atrophy. Nature Reviews. Disease Primers. 2022;**8**:56

[170] Wenning GK, Stankovic I, Vignatelli L, Fanciulli A, Calandra-Buonaura G, Seppi K, et al. The movement disorder society criteria for the diagnosis of multiple system atrophy. Journal of Movement Disorders. 2022;**37**: 1131-1148

[171] Panza F, Lozupone M, Seripa D, Daniele A, Watling M, Giannelli G, et al. Development of disease-modifying drugs for frontotemporal dementia spectrum disorders. Nature Reviews. Neurology. 2020;**16**:213-228

[172] Puppala GK, Gorthi SP, Chandran V, Gundabolu G. Frontotemporal dementia–current concepts. Neurology India. 2021;**69**:1144-1152

Section 3

Clinical Setting

Chapter 4

Neuromuscular Junction Disorders in the Elderly

Elena Shanina and Robert Glenn Smith

Abstract

The neuromuscular junction (NMJ) is unusually susceptible to disease in aging humans. Both primary autoimmune and paraneoplastic disease target the presynaptic and postsynaptic portions of the NMJ, leading to well-defined syndromes, including Lambert-Eaton myasthenic syndrome and myasthenia gravis. Primary immune disease has a bifid incidence peak, with both diseases found in younger individuals with a predilection for females and in older individuals with less or no gender specificity. Their paraneoplastic counterparts, classically identified in patients with small-cell lung carcinoma and thymomas, respectively, are much more common in older individuals. Almost 90% have onset after age 50, with 60+% of paraneoplastic disease patients being male. Although diseases of the NMJ are also diagnosed in young individuals, the lifespan of those individuals has been lengthened with available treatments, leading to specific challenges for older patients with myasthenic syndromes.

Keywords: neuromuscular junction, neuromuscular transmission, Lambert-Eaton myasthenic syndrome, myasthenia gravis, paraneoplastic disorder, thymoma, acetylcholine receptor, muscle-specific kinase, voltage-gated calcium channels, autoimmunity

1. Introduction

The two most important neuromuscular junction (NMJ) disorders in the elderly are myasthenia gravis (MG) and Lambert-Eaton myasthenic syndrome (LEMS). Both disorders are immune-mediated and can be paraneoplastic (**Table 1**). The incidence and prevalence of both diseases increase with age, with increased mortality ascribed to older afflicted individuals [1].

1.1 Muscle and neuromuscular junction in aging

Aging is associated with a slow, gradual degeneration of the NMJ, the site of synaptic connection between the motor nerve and muscle fiber, comprising the presynaptic nerve terminal, the synaptic cleft, and the specialized postsynaptic muscle endplate. Normally, when an action potential arrives at the presynaptic nerve terminal, voltage-gated calcium channels (VGCC) open at active zones with an influx of calcium, activating mobilization and release of acetylcholine (ACh) from ACh-containing vesicles. The binding of ACh to postsynaptic acetylcholine receptors

Feature	MG	LEMS
Site of pathology	Postsynaptic	Presynaptic
Antibodies involved	AChR, MuSK, LRP4	P/Q VGCC
The most common tumor when paraneoplastic	Thymoma	SCLC
Predominant site of weakness Fatigability and facilitation	Ocular, bulbar, proximal, axial Fatigable weakness, no facilitation with a short exercise	Proximal muscle Fatigable weakness, transient facilitation with a short exercise
Ocular symptoms	Common	Rare
Reflexes	Normal	Decreased or absent, Facilitated by short exercise
Dysautonomia	Absent	Present
Electrodiagnostic testing	Normal CMAP amplitude at baseline	Reduced CMAP amplitude at baseline
	Decrement of ≥10% on low-rate RNS (2–3 Hz)	Decrement of ≥10% on low-rate RNS (2–3 Hz)
	No increment on high-rate RNS (20 Hz) or short isometric exercise	Increment of 50–200% on high-rate RNS (20 Hz) or short isometric exercise
	Jitter on SFEMG	Jitter on SFEMG

Table 1.
Differences and similarities of myasthenia gravis (MG) and Lambert-Eaton myasthenic syndrome (LEMS). AChR—acetylcholine receptor, MuSK—muscle-specific kinase, LRP4—lipoprotein receptor-related protein 4, CMAP—compound motor action potential, RNS—repetitive nerve stimulation, SFEMG—single fiber electromyography, SCLC—small cell lung carcinoma, P/Q VGCC—P/Q voltage-gated calcium channel.

(AChRs) activates sodium entry through the receptor pores, causing muscle membrane depolarization and muscle contraction. However, in aged mice and in humans over age 65, morphologic remodeling presynaptically produces increased branching of nerve terminals and increased total nerve terminal branch length, number, and planar area, possibly to combat age-related decreases in terminal vesicle number and the number and concentration of active zones [2–4].

Postsynaptic changes are also observed, including increased numbers of abandoned endplate gutters, increased fragmentation of acetylcholine receptors (AChRs), decreased endplate length and area, decreased perimeter length around endplates, and increased expression of neural cell adhesion molecule (NCAM) at receptor sites [4, 5].

Depolarization of aged presynaptic junctions produces increased ACh released per vesicle, as measured electrophysiologically by increased end plate potential (EPP) size. However, with fewer vesicles per junction and increased dysfunction of presynaptic calcium entry at nerve terminal calcium channels, there is more rapid terminal exhaustion with aging, resulting in a reduced vesicle release safety factor [5].

Increased inflammatory cytokines levels, including tumor necrosis factor-alpha (TNF-alpha) and interleukin-6 (IL-6) are observed at aging junctions, which when combined with NCAM expression, increase the risk of local inflammation [6]. The increased amount of ACh released per vesicle at aging presynaptic terminals in combination with reduced agrin production produces progressive direct damage to the aging NM and increased neurotransmission failure [7].

Finally, in normal aging, the number of muscle satellite cells decreases with time, and both myotube differentiation and myosin expression in those cells decline. This leads to impaired regeneration following even minor muscle injury from exercise [8]. In addition, reduced capillary density in aging muscle further limits muscle growth and affects muscle health [9]. Satellite cells from muscle isolated from MG patients showed defective function with reduced regenerative capability [10].

Overall, these changes increase damage to aging NMJs and indirectly produce increased inflammation locally, potentially increasing immune targeting of post- or presynaptic junction sites.

1.2 Immune system and aging

With aging, T-cell receptors lose CD 28 receptor targeting and take on many cytotoxic T-cell attributes [11]. Upregulation of NCAMs, one such change, increases their targeting to inflammatory sites; these T-cells and their cytokines are expressed at much higher concentrations at inflammatory sites of patients with autoimmune diseases, suggesting their importance in autoimmune disease progression.

B-cells are the effector arm for activated T-cells, and one of the most important discovery about B cell senescence has been the recognition of populations of "age-associated B-cells" or ABCs, initially in mouse models and subsequently in humans. These B cells are of myeloid rather than lymphoid origin, and their percentage increases with age through altered transcriptional regulation. This increased ABC population inhibits the production of naïve lymphoid derived follicular B cell precursors, mediated through the release of TNF-alpha by those cells.

Overall, these ABCs appear to produce a proinflammatory microenvironment in bone marrow, inhibit survival of standard B cell precursors, and help activation of B-cell linked autoimmune disease [12].

Dysregulation of B cell repertoire in MG follows many of the same changes observed with the activation of ABCs [13]. However, it remains to be proven whether the production of autoantibodies in seropositive MG patients is derived from ABC activation as occurs in other B-cell linked autoimmune diseases [12].

Given how the aging of the NMJ and the immune system appears to increase the risk of autoimmune disease activation, the question – possibly not currently answerable - is whether there are fundamental differences in disease activation and progression between young and aged individuals with these immune diseases of the NMJ.

2. Myasthenia gravis

2.1 Epidemiology

Although myasthenia gravis is considered a rare disease, its global incidence ranges from 0.3 to 2.8 per 100,000 people, with a prevalence of approximately 10–20 per 100,000 [14, 15]. In the largest nationwide review, the rate of new diagnoses increased steadily from age 50, peaking in the 8th decade of life [16]. Testing over 30,000 newly diagnosed patients across all ages over 3 years, the reported incidence remained relatively constant at 0.3–0.5 per 100,000 person-years between ages 5–45. Thereafter, incidence rose, reaching 1.89 per 100,000 at ages 70. Hospital admission mortality rates for these patients held steady at 5.5–6.5 per 1000 between ages 10 and 40, then increased over 10-fold by the age of 80.

This increasing incidence with advanced age was initially believed to be due to better clinician ascertainment. However, this was not observed in early-onset MG [17]. The rising prevalence rates are more likely attributed to better disease management, allowing patients with MG to live longer [18].

2.2 Pathophysiology or pathogenesis

2.2.1 Antibodies and complement

Myasthenia gravis is an antibody-mediated disorder, where an immune attack targets different components of the postsynaptic membrane and causes a defect of neuromuscular transmission and fatigable weakness of skeletal muscles.

The most common antibodies (Ab) detected in patients with myasthenia gravis are anti-AChR Ab (binding, blocking, and modulating). These antibodies are mostly Ig-G1 and Ig-G3 types and are found in 80% of patients with generalized MG and 85% with ocular MG. They either directly block AChR function or bind to them causing receptor modulation - internalization with subsequent diminished potential for postsynaptic membrane activation. This process is complement-mediated, and inhibition of complement cascade at C5 reduces both AChR internalization and postsynaptic damage observed with electron microscopy.

Anti-MuSK Abs are detected in about 50% of patients seronegative for anti-AChR Ab, but they are very rare in pure ocular myasthenia. These antibodies are IgG4 class and the attack is not complement-mediated. MuSK is a protein that facilitates the clustering of AChRs, and when affected by an immune attack, reduces synaptic transmission at the NMJ.

Other antibodies more recently detected include anti-LRP4 and anti-agrin Ab, both rare and found in about 10–20% of double seronegative patients. In one large study of 635 patients, 18.7% of double seronegative patients were positive for anti-LRP4 Ab [19].

The creation of an in vivo cell-based assay (CBA) for the detection of these antibodies in their native conformation allowed most previously Ab-negative patients with MG to be identified as positive [20]. Thus, with this technique, only 1–2% of patients with MG remain as Ab-negative. Using CBAs, a recent review re-documented the superiority of this assay method in a large patient cohort over that of previously used radioimmunoprecipitation assays (RIPA) or enzyme-linked immunosorbent assays (ELISA) [21]. Note that most commercially based testing still employs these older methods of assay.

After a longstanding immune attack on the postsynaptic membrane, there are not only chemical and electrophysiologic dysfunctions reducing muscle contraction but also structural damage to the postsynaptic membrane. There, the number of postsynaptic membrane folds is reduced, with the remaining folds becoming shallower. This results in static baseline weakness in addition to fatigable weakness characteristic of patients with myasthenia. Hence, initiation of treatment before permanent structural damage occurs is paramount.

2.2.2 Cytokines and T-cells

Specific T-cell subsets are required for long-term response, and cytokines released by these T cells regulate antibody production in plasmacytes. For AChR Ab+ MG, T cells express surface inducible costimulatory (ICOS) and programmed cell death protein 1 (PD1) proteins, important for directing B-cell antibody production, and release pro-inflammatory interleukins and interferon-gamma (IFN-gamma), with suppressed IL-10 production, also important in B-cell maturation and inflammation. With immunosuppressant drug treatment, there is a reduction of IFN-gamma and upregulated IL-10 production with the conversion of TH1 to TH2 cells, reducing inflammation [22]. While significantly increased CD4 + CD28- T cell expression is observed in aging humans, these CD4 + CD28- T-cells and their cytokines are inappropriately expressed at much higher concentrations at inflammatory sites of patients with autoimmune diseases, suggesting their importance in autoimmune disease progression [23].

2.2.3 Role of thymus

The thymus is the organ responsible for developing self-tolerance and regulating the immune system. Although a role for the thymus in MG was discovered a century ago, proof that the disease was positively affected by thymic removal is relatively recent [24, 25]. With age, the thymus normally undergoes atrophy, but with MG, it is typically enlarged and contains many follicular germinal centers, like those observed in lymph nodes [26].

Overall, about 75% of MG patients have impaired thymus function, 23–35% have thymus tumors (mostly thymomas), and 65% have thymus hyperplasia [27]. It has been proposed that thymic myoepithelial cells, which express distinct nicotinic AChR subunits, may play a role in activation of thymic germinal centers.

At onset, patients with thymoma were younger than patients without thymoma (52.0 vs. 60.4 years, respectively). Clinical characteristics of MG with and without thymoma are very similar, though the disease can be more aggressive in progression when thymoma is present [28].

2.3 Diagnosis

Diagnosis of MG is made by clinical examination and special maneuvers, serological testing, and electrodiagnosis (**Table 1**).

2.3.1 Clinical evaluation

Fluctuating fatigable weakness with rapid recovery following brief rest is the hallmark of the clinical pattern of neuromuscular junction disorders [29]. In MG, patients typically report weakness by the end of the day or after a prolonged task. Affected muscles include ocular, bulbar, axial, limb (proximal more than distal, with triceps more affected than biceps), and respiratory muscles, including the diaphragm.

The most common testable symptoms of myasthenia gravis include ptosis and variable external ophthalmoplegia. These are ophthalmic signs of fatigable weakness and can be reproduced and/or measured. Cogan sign and demonstration of Hering's law of equal innervation are typical of myasthenic ptosis.

The ice-pack test is a quick, easy, safe, and affordable bedside assessment when ptosis is present. Ocular fissure is measured before the procedure, then the ice pack is applied to an affected lid, and after 2 minutes measurements are repeated. Improvement of 2 mm or more is considered diagnostic. A study of 102 patients with ocular myasthenia showed similar diagnostic accuracy of icepack test and single-fiber EMG in patients with ocular MG presenting with ptosis [30].

Non-ophthalmologic tests of fatigable bulbar weakness include single breath counting, timed sustained single breath exhalation with vowel sound, timing of onset of or worsening of dysarthria with reading aloud, and sleep testing (documenting improvement in ophthalmic and non-ophthalmic tests of weakness following a brief nap).

Muscles most prone to fatigue in MG are commonly tested for generalized fatigable weakness. These include finger extensors, elbow extensors, and hip flexors. Repetitive testing every 1–2 seconds proceeds until the patient becomes reproducibly weak in the tested muscle. Quantitation of the number of repetitions to fatigue and evidence of recovery at 2 minutes can be obtained from this testing, which has both diagnostic value and use in defining response to treatments.

Pharmacological bedside assessment (edrophonium test, neostigmine test) nowadays has limited use largely due to the need for IV access and potential cardiac side effects. However, while less dramatic, the same test can be performed in the clinic using pyridostigmine, allowing at least 30 minutes to elapse for post-ingestion testing. This test is much better tolerated by the elderly.

2.3.2 Serological testing

Due to its high sensitivity and specificity, serological testing is considered the first line of investigation. These tests can be performed simultaneously or sequentially, the latter more cost-effective but potentially causing treatment delay. When assessed sequentially, the first test to order is the anti-AChR Ab panel, assessing binding, blocking, and modulating autoantibodies. If negative, anti-MuSK Ab presence is tested, and both study panels are negative, reaction of serum against LRP4 is assessed [21]. If all studies are negative on standard tests, the reaction of patient sera to cell-based assays for conformationally sensitive epitopes on these same molecules is performed. These studies will collectively identify antibody specificity for approximately 99% of patients with myasthenia gravis. Titin and anti-striated muscle Ab occur more commonly in late-onset myasthenia and are associated with severe disease.

2.3.3 Electrodiagnostic testing

Repetitive nerve stimulation (RNS) is usually performed when serological testing is negative, equivocal, or unavailable. Low-rate stimulation at 2–3 Hz causes no change in compound motor action potential (CMAP) amplitude in normal individuals due to the vesicular release (quantal transmission) safety factor. In MG, this safety factor is reduced, producing post-synaptic exhaustion of transmission at this same rate of repetitive stimulation, leading to reduced CMAP amplitude following each stimulation in the test train. When the test is properly administered, a CMAP decrement of 10% between the first and fourth pulses in the train is considered diagnostic for neuromuscular junction transmission defect. To increase the sensitivity of the test, isometric exercise is usually performed, with postexercise decrement measurements. Clinically weak or fatigable muscles should undergo this testing, which is challenging in pure ocular myasthenia.

In an inpatient setting, RNS is more rapidly available compared to serological testing and a recent study showed high sensitivity and specificity in patients requiring hospitalization [31].

Single-fiber EMG is considered the most sensitive method for documenting the presence of neuromuscular junction disorders, but it requires highly trained specialists, usually in tertiary neuromuscular centers, and is not readily available. When a pair of two motor unit action potentials are collected, the first potential is time-locked, and when abnormal, the second shows increased variability of response time (jitter) and impulse blocking. When positive, this test indicates defective neuromuscular transmission and in most MG patients, correlates with disease severity and clinical course [32].

2.3.4 Imaging

A chest CT with contrast is the study of choice and is recommended at the time of diagnosis, to exclude the presence of paraneoplastic MG due to thymoma. Results can include not only the detection of a tumor but evidence of thymic hyperplasia, though rare in the aging population compared to the young. If initially negative, the CT chest is often repeated after one to 2 years, especially if the disease is difficult to control. If positive for tumor, 90% of thymomas are benign, but evidence for rapid tumor removal eventually improving or completely "curing" the patient's MG is overwhelming. Once removed, however, thymoma surveillance should continue. The National Comprehensive Cancer Network (NCCN) recommends conducting surveillance chest CT every 6 months for 2 years and then annually for 10 years [33].

2.3.5 Diagnostic challenges in the elderly population

Diagnostic challenges and substantial underdiagnosis of elderly individuals with MG can be explained by comorbid diseases masking the diagnosis. Many of the presenting symptoms of MG, including dysarthria, dysphagia, muscle weakness, and fatigue have a broad differential diagnosis in older individuals and are often attributed to stroke and other central nervous system disorders. Aging also causes lid sagging, masking the ability to detect ptosis from MG. Diplopia may be difficult to determine because of reduced vision from cataracts or macular degeneration. Limb weakness and dyspnea may be attributed to comorbid cardiac disease, pulmonary disease, or deconditioning, and recovery from fatigue may be slower secondary to comorbid disease and age-dependent AChR complex degeneration. All United Kingdom Centers national AChR Ab incidence studies showed high detection of seropositivity in previously unrecognized patients in patients >75 years old [34].

Most patients in the 65+ age range have initial ocular symptoms rapidly progressing to generalized disease and had an initially aggressive course [35]. In patients >85, early mortality was over 10% [16]. However, increased morbidity and mortality were primarily seen in patients who were not placed immediately on immunotherapy [29].

2.4 Classifications

Myasthenia gravis can be classified based on clinical manifestations, severity, serological status, and age of onset.

Ocular myasthenia defined by isolated fatigable weakness of ocular muscles (ptosis, diplopia, eye closure weakness), represents only 15% of patients. Generalized myasthenia can involve limb, axial, bulbar, and respiratory muscles.

The clinical severity of MG is assessed by the Myasthenia Gravis Foundation of America (MGFA) classification as Classes I-V. Class I is defined as isolated ocular muscle weakness, Classes II-IV as mild, moderate, and severe weakness involving other muscles respectively, and Class V when respiratory failure requires intubation [36].

Seropositive patients have one of the respective antibodies: anti-AChR+MG, anti-MuSK+MG, anti-LRP4 + MG. Seronegative MG is classified in patients without detectable antibodies. In such cases, the diagnosis is confirmed by other tests.

It is important to determine serological status and what type of antibodies each patient has, as this might determine the clinical course and response to treatment. Patients with late-onset of the disease have a higher proportion of anti-AChR+MG.

Early-onset MG corresponds to the presentation before the age of 50. There is female predominance, and thymic hyperplasia is common. Late-onset MG is defined as the onset of 50 years or older. Both genders are affected with a slightly higher prevalence of males after the age of 60. Thymic hyperplasia is absent after age 65.

About 50% of patients with thymoma have AChR antibodies and about 30–40% develop clinical manifestations of MG. Conversely, about 10–20% of patients with MG have thymus tumors. Thymoma can develop at any age, with a reported mean age of 52.

2.4.1 Relation to immune checkpoint inhibitor use

Immune checkpoint inhibitors (ICI) have an increasing role in advanced cancer management supported by improved survival and longer remissions. Checkpoint proteins expressed on cancer cells prevent normal autoimmunity and, thus allow cancer cells to be missed from a normal antitumor immune response. However, while ICIs can activate the immune system against cancer, they may also trigger autoimmune diseases.

ICI-related MG can occur as de novo disease or exacerbation of the preexisting MG. These immune adverse events are relatively rare but result in severe morbidity and fatalities. Most patients develop MG symptoms within a median of 4 weeks after initiation of ICI treatment, 63–83% develop rapidly progressive moderate to severe weakness, about 50% require mechanical ventilation and the mortality rate reaches 30%. Elevated AChR antibodies were noted in 66% of patients and none had thymoma [37]. In some cases, ICI-related MG coexists with myositis and myocarditis ("3 M triad").

Likely due to targeted populations for ICI treatments, most patients are elderly males with a median age of 73 years.

Currently, there are several classes of ICI targeting antibodies against: programmed cell death-1 (PD-1) receptors (pembrolizumab, nivolumab, cemiplimab), programmed cell death-ligand 1 (PD-L1) (atezolizumab, avelumab, durvalumab), cytotoxic T-lymphocyte-associated antigen-4 (CTLA-4) (ipilimumab, tremelimumab), and lymphocyte-activation gene 3 (LG3) (relatlimab). Most reported cases received anti-PD-1 therapy or a combination of different ICIs.

Early initiation of rescue treatment with IV Immunoglobulin (IVIG) or plasmapheresis regardless of disease severity showed better outcomes, than steroids [37]. Rituximab, cyclophosphamide, and azathioprine have been reported effective for long-term treatment. ICI is usually stopped while acute treatment of induced MG is conducted. The decision to continue ICI treatment is based on the individual case and successful rechallenge with a different agent or a different class ICI has been reported.

2.5 Treatment

Currently there is no cure for MG, however, management has significantly improved in recent years. Treatment options include symptomatic and

Treatment type/ mechanism	Common medications	Route	Onset of effect	Type of MG
Symptomatic, AChE inhibition	Pyridostigmine	PO	30–60 min	Any
Corticosteroids	Prednisone	PO	<3 weeks	Any
Common steroid-sparing agents	Azathioprine	PO	6–18 months	Any
	Mycophenolate mofetil	PO	3–12 months	Any
	Cyclosporine	PO	1–3 months	Any
	Tacrolimus	PO	1–6 months	Any
	Methotrexate	PO	6–12 months	Any
	Cyclophosphamide	PO	1–6 months	Any
B-cell inhibitors	Rituximab	IV	1–3 months	MuSK+and refractory gMG
Complement inhibitors	Eculizumab	IV	1–4 weeks	AChR+ gMG
	Ravulizumab	IV	1–4 weeks	AChR+ gMG
	Zilucoplan		1–4 weeks	AChR+ gMG
FcRN receptor inhibitors	Efgartigimod	IV/SQ	<2 weeks	AChR+ gMG
	Rosanolixumab	SQ	<2 weeks	AChR+, MuSK+ gMG
IVIG	Immunoglobulin	IV	3–10 days	gMG
SCIG	Immunoglobulin	SQ	<2 weeks	gMG
Plasma exchange	Plasma exchange	IV	2–5 days	gMG
Thymectomy		Robotic surgery	12–18 months	Thymoma associated, AchR+

Table 2.
Summary of current treatment options for myasthenia gravis (MG). AChE—acetylcholine esterase, gMG—generalized myasthenia gravis, AChR+—acetylcholine receptor seropositive, MuSK+—muscle-specific kinase seropositive.

immunomodulating (**Table 2**). The choice of treatment depends on balancing disease severity, serological type, comorbidities, and quality of life in therapeutic intervention decisions.

2.5.1 Acetylcholine esterase inhibitors (AChEI)

The cornerstone of MG symptomatic treatment is the use of AChEIs. They improve neuromuscular transmission at the motor endplate by slowing ACh degradation and prolonging its effects. They are very effective and can be sufficient for treating mild symptomatic disease, though they have no actual effect on disease suppression. Pyridostigmine bromide is the most used AChEI worldwide. Side effects include diarrhea, increased bronchial secretions, and hypersalivation, and they should be used only as necessary in chronic therapy of late-onset disease [38] because of their indirect effects on worsening NMJ degradation in the elderly. For these reasons, primary immunomodulatory therapy needs to accompany symptomatic treatment in all patients with late-onset MG (> 65 years).

2.5.2 Plasmapheresis and immunoglobulin

Both plasmapheresis and intravenous immunoglobulin (IVIG) are reserved for the management of myasthenic crisis, acute exacerbation, refractory course and preoperative management of MG [36]. IVIg should be administered with caution in patients over 65 years and patients with a history of cardiac and cerebrovascular diseases, secondary to their effects on serum viscosity, thromboembolism, vasospasm, worsening hypertension, and renal injury. Many clinicians slow the rate of IVIg administration by 50% in older patients to reduce the risk of these side effects [39].

Subcutaneous immunoglobulin (SCIg) is far more difficult for elderly patients to master since it requires self-injection via a pump. When caregivers of older patients or physically stronger patients can perform the procedure, however, it bypasses the need for separate IV access and does not increase serum viscosity [40].

The benefits of plasma exchange in treating MG have been known for almost half a century. However, access to an apheresis center limits care for many patients. Early response to therapy is often best observed using this modality, especially in myasthenic crises.

2.5.3 Corticosteroids

Corticosteroids are very effective and can be used in all MG types. They were among the first immunotherapies available for MG and are still almost universally used in its initial treatment. Although disease remission can be achieved within a few weeks of treatment, a slow ramping dose is recommended to prevent initial deterioration with drug initiation. Further, chronic side effects of steroid therapy at therapeutic doses include steroid-induced diabetes, osteoporosis, hypertension, weight gain, infections, and rapid cataract formation [41].

2.5.4 Steroid-sparing immunosuppressive agents

Azathioprine, a purine synthesis cytotoxic antimetabolite, is the most used steroid-sparing immunosuppressive agent for the long-term management of MG worldwide. It is effective and generally well tolerated by patients, but therapeutic onset is delayed and takes 6–18 months to achieve therapeutic benefit. Therefore, it is often started together with steroids. However, in elderly patients with good hepatic function, who are not taking allopurinol or warfarin, it is usually well tolerated [42].

Other oral steroid-sparing agents include mycophenolate mofetil - a potent monophosphate dehydrogenase inhibitor and methotrexate – a folate antimetabolite. Though initially controversial in MG treatment, both treatments have more recently been shown to be efficacious – with methotrexate more rapidly effective in treating aggressive disease [43, 44]. Cyclosporine A – a calcineurin inhibitor – is not recommended for patients with late-onset disease because of its deleterious and often permanent effects on renal function. Tacrolimus is also a calcineurin inhibitor and is effective in treating MG. It has less nephrotoxicity than cyclosporine but has a dose-dependent and reversible side effect of tremor, and a less reversible side effect of sensory polyneuropathy, both problematic in older patients [45].

2.5.5 Complement inhibitors

Anti-AChR Ab belong to complement-fixing subclasses (IgG1 and IgG3) and their pathogenicity is in part due to complement system activation. Blockade of complement activation at several steps can prevent membrane attack complex formation and post-synaptic endplate membrane lysis. At present, prevention of C5 cleavage is the preferred treatment to block complement-mediated membrane damage. Because complement is involved in AChR Ab-mediated attacks, and not in MuSK or LRP4 antibodies (IgG4 subclass), only patients with AChR Ab+ MG are candidates for this treatment [46, 47].

The first human complement C5 inhibitor approved for MG, Eculizumab, is a humanized monoclonal antibody that binds with high affinity to terminal complement C5 with infusions every 2 weeks [47]. The first long-acting C5 complement inhibitor, ravulizumab, was engineered from eculizumab with a longer half-life, maintaining therapeutic serum concentrations over 8-week period [48]. The first subcutaneous form of C5 inhibitor, zilucoplan, is a targeted peptide with once-daily self-administered injections. Unlike monoclonal antibodies, this medication can be co-administered with IVIG and PLEX in severe cases [46].

Pre-vaccination to protect against encapsulated bacterial infections – primarily meningococcal infections – is necessary before beginning anti-complement therapies.

2.5.6 Neonatal Fc receptor (FcRN) inhibitors

The FcRN is important in IgG recycling. Blocking FcRN receptors promotes IgG catabolism and therefore reduces total circulating IgG, including pathological MG autoantibodies [49, 50].

The first FcRN antagonist approved for myasthenia gravis, efgartigimod, is available in both intravenous and subcutaneous forms, this drug is currently only approved for AChR Ab+ disease but should be effective against all antibody-targeted forms of MG [51]. Rosanolixizumab, another FcRN inhibitor, is administered subcutaneously and is the first in this class approved for anti-MuSK Ab+ MG [52]. Several other "me too" medications in this class are currently in clinical trials, including Nipocalimab and Batoclimab [50].

2.5.7 Prospective targets and emerging treatments

Emerging genetically engineered cell therapies include Chimeric Ag receptor T (CART) CART cell therapy and chimeric autoantibody receptor T (CAART) cell therapy are currently under investigation for generalized MG [53, 54].

Autologous hematopoietic stem cell transplant (HSCT) has been studied in a small group of patients with refractory MG and showed promising results with the achievement of remission and freedom from any MG therapy in all patients [55]. A future prospective study is warranted.

2.5.8 Surgical management

Thymectomy is indicated in patients with thymoma. Many patients with MG without thymoma who have ACR Ab also benefit from thymectomy, particularly with thymus hyperplasia. However, there is limited data on the elderly population.

An international randomized clinical trial (MGTX trial) showed the superiority of transsternal thymectomy in non-thymomatous MG patients compared to prednisone alone, but the age ceiling in this trial was 65 years, with only a small number of participants over the age of 50 [24]. In recent years open transsternal access has been replaced by video-assisted thoracoscopic surgery (VATS) and robot-assisted thoracic surgery (RATS), significantly reducing the risk of surgical morbidity [56].

Older individuals with MG without thymoma are less likely to be treated with thymectomy due to common practice and clinical guidelines, although clinical trial data is lacking [57].

3. Lambert-Eaton myasthenic syndrome

3.1 Epidemiology

Lambert-Eaton myasthenic syndrome (LEMS) is less than one 10th as prevalent as MG (2.7–7.5/1,000,000). It was first described as a separate syndrome by Edward Lambert and Lee Eaton in 1957, initially recognized as a largely paraneoplastic syndrome [58, 59]. However, like MG, it is mostly a disease of aging. More than 50% of patients with LEMS have small-cell lung carcinoma (SCLC) [59, 60], though other tumors (other lung cancers, renal cell carcinoma, lymphoproliferative tumors, prostate cancer, thymomas) are implicated in the syndrome in an additional 10–15% [58–60]. LEMS symptoms often precede identification of cancer by as much as 5 years [61]. Historical risks for paraneoplastic LEMS include weight loss, being male, and a history of smoking. The mean age of paraneoplastic disease onset is 67+/−9 years in several studies and is predominantly male [60, 62].

.The remaining patients have non-tumor-associated disease (NT-LEMS). The mean NT-LEMS age of onset – previously reported as 35 years –in a more recent study with more complete population ascertainment has been reported as 57+/−11 years [60]. While the lifespan of patients with paraneoplastic disease is dependent on the associated cancer, NT-LEMS survival is not different from the unaffected population [63]. Early differentiation between paraneoplastic and non-paraneoplastic LEMS has been reported even in the absence of direct cancer identification through the presence of antibodies to a highly immunogenic tumor antigen – SOX-1 - associated with SCLC-LEMS and other paraneoplastic syndromes (present in 64% of patients with SCLC-LEMS and in no patients with NT-LEMS).

3.2 Pathophysiology

Summarizing decades of research in a few sentences, the neurophysiologic, biochemical, and ultrastructural correlate of motor facilitation is the targeting of presynaptic P/Q voltage-gated calcium channels (VGCC) by specific antibodies, blocking or reducing calcium entry and subsequently the size and number of readily releasable neurotransmitter vesicles at presynaptic release sites [64]. This leads to reduced transmitter release and reduced post-synaptic quanta documented electrophysiologically, often to the point that the miniature endplate potential (MEPP) density is insufficient to produce muscle contraction. With brief maximal exercise, enough calcium enters presynaptically so that the readily releasable vesical pool is more easily activated. This results in increased transmitter release, increased post-synaptic MEPP density, and increased muscle action potential firing with muscle contraction [65]. However, because the vesicle pool is reduced at release sites, subsequent loss of vesicle release and motor fatigue ensues.

The presence of anti-P/Q VGCC Ab is eventually observed in over 90% of LEMS patients, and these antibodies when transferred to a mouse model reproduce the disease clinically, electrophysiologically, and morphologically [66]. Thus, these antibodies, like those observed in MG, are directly pathologic, and not simply markers for a disease type. Still, titers of these antibodies in patient serum do not directly coordinate with disease severity.

In addition to targeting the P/Q VGCC at the neuromuscular junction, there is suspected overlap to presynaptic cholinergic autonomic nerve release sites, to produce the findings of dysautonomia seen in so many patients with LEMS [67, 68]. Further, the targeting of VGCCs and of calcium release has long term affects at the NMJ structurally, noted by the dysregulation of readily releasable vesicle sites on the presynaptic membrane. Laminin beta2, found in the NMJ, binds to the P/Q type VGCC responsible for neurotransmitter release from motor nerve terminals [69]. This interaction leads to the clustering of VGCCs, which in turn recruits other presynaptic components. Perturbation of this interaction in animal models by VGCC Ab results in disassembly of ACh release sites, resembling defects observed in LEMS.

3.3 Clinical symptoms and diagnosis

The classic triad of clinical symptoms includes proximal muscle weakness – most significantly affecting hip flexors and knee extensors, decreased tendon reflexes, and autonomic dysfunction [70]. Although respiratory failure is almost never a presenting or early symptom of LEMS, unlike MG, rare patients who do die from LEMS often have late-onset respiratory dysfunction contributing to their demise. Dysarthria, dysphagia, diplopia, and ptosis, likewise observed in later disease, are generally significantly milder than observed in patients with MG [71].

Several clinical findings may distinguish LEMS from MG (**Table 1**). In patients with paraneoplastic disease, about 10% of patients show cerebellar signs, consistent with other paraneoplastic antibody-targeted disease [59, 72]. And although not common as an early finding, eventually symptoms of dysautonomia are observed in over 75% of affected individuals [70, 72]. These include xerostomia and/or xerophthalmia, hyper- or hypohydrosis, orthostatic hypotension, impotence, or abnormal pupillary response to light. Painful myalgias may also be observed in a third of patients in association with fatigue, not present in most patients with MG.

Patients with LEMS may also complain of weakness greater than can be identified clinically [71]. Early in their disease, most patients discover that although initially weak, if they give full effort for a few seconds, maximal voluntary contraction will transiently improve muscle function. Because of the combination of exercise-induced facilitation – a finding specific to LEMS – and muscle fatiguability, described clinical symptoms are often worse than observed clinical signs.

Clinical demonstration of facilitation is a hallmark of this disease [73]. This can be observed in over half of LEMS patients by documenting the difference between baseline at-rest motor strength, and muscle function after 10 seconds of maximal motor activity. Facilitation also can be observed with changes in initially reduced or absent deep tendon reflexes pre- and post-muscle activity.

Diagnosis is made on the basis of the appropriate clinical history and examination, positive serology for P/Q type VGCCs, and electromyography, documenting facilitation electrophysiologically.

3.4 Treatment

Management of paraneoplastic LEMS is directed more to reduce disease symptoms than to prolong survival – the latter dependent on the type of tumor that triggers the immune-mediated disease. Interestingly, both the presence of LEMS symptoms before identification of the instigating tumor and the increased survival of patients with SCLC with paraneoplastic LEMS relative to SCLC alone suggest that the presence of paraneoplastic disease is likely bystander injury associated with superior immune targeting of the tumor by the host [72]. Treatment of these patients with immunomodulatory therapies does not reduce cancer survival, even though they reduce the sequelae of the immune disease.

For symptomatic management of paraneoplastic and NT-LEMS, agents that enhance presynaptic acetylcholine release, like guanidine hydrochloride and 4-aminopyridine, can be effective but are typically associated with significant neurological side effects. A related compound, 3,4- diaminopyridine, acts peripherally as a depolarizing agent at the motor nerve terminal by blocking potassium efflux, thereby increasing calcium entry and enhancing quantal neurotransmitter release. This medication has far fewer side effects and is effective in reducing weakness and fatigue symptoms [70]. 3,4-diaminopyridine, under the name of amifampridine, is FDA-approved for the treatment of LEMS. Like MG symptomatic treatment, pyridostigmine is useful in increasing ACh at the NMJ and has some effects on reducing motor fatigue. The combination is more effective symptomatically than either treatment alone [63].

While standard immunomodulatory medications have been used to treat LEMS, the rarity of the disease limits data collection on the efficacy of those treatments. Nonetheless, azathioprine, mycophenolate mofetil, prednisone, and rituximab have all been reported to have long-term benefits in NT LEMS control in a single case or small uncontrolled studies [74, 75]. Plasmapheresis and IVIG have reported short-term benefits on patient symptoms with LEMS, just as observed for patients with other antibody-mediated immune diseases.

4. Conclusions

The neuromuscular junction (NMJ) disorders are a group of conditions that affect the transmission of signals between nerves and muscles, leading to fatigable muscle weakness. These disorders, while rare, become increasingly frequent with age. Conditions such as MG and LEMS are autoimmune and can be paraneoplastic, necessitating thorough examinations and often tumor treatments. As individuals age, changes occur at the NMJ and immune system that further contribute to neuromuscular dysfunction and may predispose to these disorders.

Several challenges are specific to elderly populations. These include delayed diagnosis, comorbid conditions, polypharmacy, increased risk of falls, slower response to treatment, and mobility issues. Elderly individuals often have multiple health conditions that can mask the clinical picture and delay diagnosis of NMJ disorders. They also can require complicated management, leading to polypharmacy with the potential for drug interactions and even medication-related neuromuscular transmission failure. Older patients are more likely to have paraneoplastic disease, or to receive immunotherapy for advanced cancers, including immune checkpoint inhibitors, which are known to cause drug-induced MG. Late onset LEMS is more often

DOI: http://dx.doi.org/10.5772/intechopen.1007348

associated with small cell lung cancer. Simultaneous management of malignancy and an autoimmune NMJ disorder is complex, requiring appropriate expertise.

Fatigable weakness related to NMJ disorders has profound impacts on mobility and quality of life in elderly population. It increases risk for falls and related injuries. Dysarthria and dysphagia can lead to poor communication and difficulties expressing concerns and malnutrition.

While NMJ disorders cannot yet be cured, advancements in treatment have led to significant overall clinical improvement, with many patients experiencing minimal symptoms or disease stabilization. Therefore, early recognition and initiation of treatment are critical. The rapid growth of therapeutic modalities brings new opportunities for improved quality of life and, improved survival.

Author details

Elena Shanina[1]* and Robert Glenn Smith[2]

1 University of Texas Medical Branch, Galveston, USA

2 Houston Methodist Hospital, Houston, USA

*Address all correspondence to: elshanin@utmb.edu

References

[1] Grob D, Brunner N, Namba T, Pagala M. Lifetime course of myasthenia gravis. Muscle and Nerve. 2008;**37**(2):141-149

[2] Khosa S, Trikamji B, Khosa GS, Khanli HM, Mishra SK. An overview of neuromuscular junction aging findings in human and animal studies. Current Aging Science. 2019;**12**(1):28-34

[3] Deschenes MR, Wilson MH. Age-related differences in synaptic plasticity following muscle unloading. Journal of Neurobiology. 2003;**57**(3):246-256

[4] Deschenes MR, Flannery R, Hawbaker A, Patek L, Mifsud M. Adaptive remodeling of the neuromuscular junction with aging. Cells. 2022;**11**(7):1150

[5] Iyer SR, Shah SB, Lovering RM. The neuromuscular junction: Roles in aging and neuromuscular disease. International Journal of Molecular Sciences. 2021;**22**(15):8058

[6] Fulop T, Larbi A, Pawelec G, Khalil A, Cohen AA, Hirokawa K, et al. Immunology of aging: The birth of inflammaging. Clinical Reviews in Allergy and Immunology. 2021;**64**(2):109-122

[7] Arnold WD, Clark BC. Neuromuscular junction transmission failure in aging and sarcopenia: The nexus of the neurological and muscular systems. Ageing Research Reviews. 2023;**89**:101966

[8] Hwang AB, Brack AS. Muscle stem cells and aging. Current Topics in Developmental Biology. 2018;**126**:299-322. DOI: 10.1016/bs.ctdb.2017.08.008

[9] Englund DA, Zhang X, Aversa Z, LeBrasseur NK. Skeletal muscle aging, cellular senescence, and senotherapeutics: Current knowledge and future directions. Mechanisms of Ageing and Development. 2021;**200**:111595

[10] Attia M, Maurer M, Robinet M, Le Grand F, Fadel E, Le Panse R, et al. Muscle satellite cells are functionally impaired in myasthenia gravis: Consequences on muscle regeneration. Acta Neuropathologica. 2017;**134**(6):869-888

[11] Pereira BI, De Maeyer RPH, Covre LP, Nehar-Belaid D, Lanna A, Ward S, et al. Sestrins induce natural killer function in senescent-like CD8+ T cells. Nature Immunology. 2020;**21**(6):684-694

[12] Mouat IC, Goldberg E, Horwitz MS. Age-associated B cells in autoimmune diseases. Cellular and Molecular Life Sciences. 2022;**79**(8):402

[13] Vander Heiden JA, Stathopoulos P, Zhou JQ, Chen L, Gilbert TJ, Bolen CR, et al. Dysregulation of B cell repertoire formation in myasthenia gravis patients revealed through deep sequencing. The Journal of Immunology. 2017;**198**(4):1460-1473

[14] Engebretsen I, Gilhus NE, Kristiansen IS, Sæther EM, Lindberg-Schager I, Arneberg F, et al. The epidemiology and societal costs of myasthenia gravis in Norway: A non-interventional study using national registry data. European Journal of Neurology. 2024;**31**(5):e16233

[15] Gilhus NE, Tzartos S, Evoli A, Palace J, Burns TM, Verschuuren JJGM. Myasthenia gravis. Nature Reviews Disease Primers (Nature Publishing Group). 2019;**5**(1):30. DOI: 10.1038/s41572-019-0079-y

[16] Chen J, Tian DC, Zhang C, Li Z, Zhai Y, Xiu Y, et al. Incidence, mortality, and economic burden of myasthenia gravis in China: A nationwide population-based study. The Lancet Regional Health – Western Pacific. 2020;**5**:100063. DOI: 10.1016/j.lanwpc.2020.100063

[17] Alkhawajah NM, Oger J. Late-onset myasthenia gravis: A review when incidence in older adults keeps increasing. Muscle & Nerve. 2013;**48**(5):705-710

[18] Breiner A, Widdifield J, Katzberg HD, Barnett C, Bril V, Tu K. Epidemiology of myasthenia gravis in Ontario, Canada. Neuromuscular Disorders. 2016;**26**(1):41-46

[19] Zisimopoulou P, Evangelakou P, Tzartos J, Lazaridis K, Zouvelou V, Mantegazza R, et al. A comprehensive analysis of the epidemiology and clinical characteristics of anti-LRP4 in myasthenia gravis. Journal of Autoimmunity. 2014;**52**:139-145

[20] Vincent A, Waters P, Leite MI, Jacobson L, Koneczny I, Cossins J, et al. Antibodies identified by cell-based assays in myasthenia gravis and associated diseases. Annals of the New York Academy of Sciences. 2012;**1274**:92-98

[21] Li Y, Peng Y, Yang H. Serological diagnosis of myasthenia gravis and its clinical significance. Annals of Translational Medicine. 2023;**11**(7):290

[22] Çebi M, Durmus H, Aysal F, Özkan B, Gül GE, Çakar A, et al. CD4+ T cells of myasthenia gravis patients are characterized by increased IL-21, IL-4, and IL-17A productions and higher presence of PD-1 and ICOS. Frontiers in Immunology. 2020;**11**:809

[23] Wang L, Wang FS, Gershwin ME. Human autoimmune diseases: A comprehensive update. Journal of Internal Medicine. 2015;**278**(4):369-395

[24] Wolfe GI, Kaminski HJ, Aban IB, Minisman G, Kuo HC, Marx A, et al. Randomized trial of thymectomy in myasthenia gravis. New England Journal of Medicine. 2016;**375**(6):511-522

[25] Menon D, Barnett C, Bril V. Novel treatments in myasthenia gravis. Frontiers in Neurology. 2020;**11**:538

[26] Truffault F, de Montpreville V, Eymard B, Sharshar T, Le Panse R, Berrih-Aknin S. Thymic germinal centers and corticosteroids in myasthenia gravis: An immunopathological study in 1035 cases and a critical review. Clinical Reviews in Allergy and Immunology. 2017;**52**(1):108-124

[27] Suzuki T, Hishida T, Suzuki S, Okubo Y, Masai K, Kaseda K, et al. Clinicopathological predictors of postoperative long-term myasthenic status in resected thymoma with myasthenia gravis. Surgery Today. 2024;**54**(7):787-794

[28] Álvarez-Velasco R, Gutiérrez-Gutiérrez G, Trujillo JC, Martínez E, Segovia S, Arribas-Velasco M, et al. Clinical characteristics and outcomes of thymoma-associated myasthenia gravis. European Journal of Neurology. 2021;**28**(6):2083-2091

[29] Cortés-Vicente E, Álvarez-Velasco R, Segovia S, Paradas C, Casasnovas C, Guerrero-Sola A, et al. Clinical and therapeutic features of myasthenia gravis in adults based on age at onset. Neurology. 2020;**94**(11):e1171-e1180

[30] Giannoccaro MP, Paolucci M, Zenesini C, Di Stasi V, Donadio V, Avoni P, et al. Comparison of ice pack test and single-fiber EMG diagnostic accuracy in patients referred for

myasthenic ptosis. Neurology. 2020;**95**(13):E1800-E1806

[31] Clifford KM, Wu CK, Post D, Shaik R, Muppidi S. Utility of repetitive nerve stimulation in the diagnosis of myasthenia gravis in the inpatient setting. Neurohospitalist. 2023;**13**(4):364-370

[32] Baruca M, Leonardis L, Podnar S, Hojs-Fabjan T, Grad A, Jerin A, et al. Single fiber EMG as a prognostic tool in myasthenia gravis. Muscle & Nerve. 2016;**54**(6):1034-1040

[33] Strange CD, Ahuja J, Shroff GS, Truong MT, Marom EM. Imaging evaluation of thymoma and thymic carcinoma. Frontiers in Oncology. 2021;**11**:810419

[34] Vincent A, Clover L, Buckley C, Evans G, Rothwell PM. Evidence of underdiagnosis of myasthenia gravis in older people. Journal of Neurology, Neurosurgery, and Psychiatry. 2003;**74**(8):1105-1108

[35] Tang YL, Ruan Z, Su Y, Guo RJ, Gao T, Liu Y, et al. Clinical characteristics and prognosis of very late-onset myasthenia gravis in China. Neuromuscular Disorders. 2023;**33**(4):358-366

[36] Jaretzki A, Barohn RJ, Ernstoff RM, Kaminski HJ, Keesey JC, Penn AS, et al. Myasthenia gravis: Recommendations for clinical research standards. Neurology. 2000;**55**(1):16-23

[37] Safa H, Johnson DH, Trinh VA, Rodgers TE, Lin H, Suarez-Almazor ME, et al. Immune checkpoint inhibitor related myasthenia gravis: Single center experience and systematic review of the literature. Journal for Immunotherapy of Cancer. 2019;**7**(1):319

[38] Punga AR, Sawada M, Stålberg EV. Electrophysiological signs and the prevalence of adverse effects of acetylcholinesterase inhibitors in patients with myasthenia gravis. Muscle & Nerve. 2008;**37**(3):300-307

[39] Ammann EM, Haskins CB, Fillman KM, Ritter RL, Gu X, Winiecki SK, et al. Intravenous immune globulin and thromboembolic adverse events: A systematic review and meta-analysis of RCTs. American Journal of Hematology. 2016;**91**(6):594-605

[40] Sala TP, Crave JC, Duracinsky M, Lepira Bompeka F, Tadmouri A, Chassany O, et al. Efficacy and patient satisfaction in the use of subcutaneous immunoglobulin immunotherapy for the treatment of auto-immune neuromuscular diseases. Autoimmunity Reviews. 2018;**17**:873-881

[41] Alkhawajah NM, Oger J. Treatment of myasthenia gravis in the aged. Drugs & Aging. 2015;**32**(9):689-697

[42] Moura J, Fernandes J, Lima MJ, Sousa AP, Samões R, Martins Silva A, et al. Treatment strategies and treatment-related adverse events in MG according to the age of onset. Frontiers in Neurology [Internet]. 2024;**15**:1277420. Available from: http://www.ncbi.nlm.nih.gov/pubmed/38529037 [Accessed: July 6, 2024]

[43] Narayanaswami P, Sanders DB, Thomas L, Thibault D, Blevins J, Desai R, et al. Comparative Effectiveness of Azathioprine and Mycophenolate Mofetil for Myasthenia Gravis (PROMISE-MG): A Prospective Cohort Study [Internet]. 2024. Available from: www.thelancet.com/neurology

[44] Dodd KC, Ahmed R, Ambrose P, Holt JK, Jacob S, Leite MI, et al. Mycophenolate and methotrexate are better tolerated than azathioprine in myasthenia gravis. Neuromuscular Disorders. 2024;**38**:51-57

[45] Fan Z, Li Z, Shen F, Zhang X, Lei L, Su S, et al. Favorable effects of tacrolimus monotherapy on myasthenia gravis patients. Frontiers in Neurology. 2020;**11**:594152

[46] Weiss MD, Bresch S, Freimer M, Hewamadduma C, Juntas-Morales R, Leite MI, et al. Subgroup outcomes from RAISE: A randomized, phase 3 trial of zilucoplan in generalized myasthenia gravis (P1-5.006). Neurology. 2023;**100**(17_Suppl. 2):2940

[47] Howard JF, Utsugisawa K, Benatar M, Murai H, Barohn RJ, Illa I, et al. Safety and efficacy of eculizumab in anti-acetylcholine receptor antibody-positive refractory generalised myasthenia gravis (REGAIN): A phase 3, randomised, double-blind, placebo-controlled, multicentre study. Lancet Neurology. 2017;**16**(12):976-986

[48] Vu T, Meisel A, Mantegazza R, Annane D, Katsuno M, Aguzzi R, et al. Terminal complement inhibitor ravulizumab in generalized myasthenia gravis. NEJM Evidence. 2022;**1**(5):EVIDoa2100066

[49] Dalakas MC, Spaeth PJ. The importance of FcRn in neuro-immunotherapies: From IgG catabolism, FCGRT gene polymorphisms, IVIg dosing and efficiency to specific FcRn inhibitors. Therapeutic Advances in Neurological Disorders. 2021;**14**:1756286421997381

[50] Bhandari V, Bril V. FcRN receptor antagonists in the management of myasthenia gravis. Frontiers in Neurology. 2023;**14**:1229112

[51] Howard JF, Bril V, Vu T, Karam C, Peric S, Margania T, et al. Safety, efficacy, and tolerability of efgartigimod in patients with generalised myasthenia gravis (ADAPT): A multicentre, randomised, placebo-controlled, phase 3 trial. Lancet Neurology. 2021;**20**(7):526-536

[52] Bril V, Drużdż A, Grosskreutz J, Habib AA, Mantegazza R, Sacconi S, et al. Safety and efficacy of rozanolixizumab in patients with generalised myasthenia gravis (MycarinG): A randomised, double-blind, placebo-controlled, adaptive phase 3 study. Lancet Neurology. 2023;**22**(5):383-394

[53] Granit V, Benatar M, Kurtoglu M, Miljković MD, Chahin N, Sahagian G, et al. Safety and clinical activity of autologous RNA chimeric antigen receptor T-cell therapy in myasthenia gravis (MG-001): A prospective, multicentre, open-label, non-randomised phase 1b/2a study. Lancet Neurology. 2023;**22**(7):578-590

[54] Oh S, Payne AS. Engineering cell therapies for autoimmune diseases: From preclinical to clinical proof of concept. Immune Network. 2022;**22**(5):e37

[55] Bryant A, Atkins H, Pringle CE, Allan D, Anstee G, Bence-Bruckler I, et al. Myasthenia gravis treated with autologous hematopoietic stem cell transplantation. JAMA Neurology. 2016;**73**(6):652-658

[56] Shen C, Li J, Li J, Che G. Robot-assisted thoracic surgery versus video-assisted thoracic surgery for treatment of patients with thymoma: A systematic review and meta-analysis. Thoracic Cancer. 2022;**13**(2):151-161

[57] Morganroth J, Zuroff L, Guidon AC, Liu GT, Bird SJ, Singhal S, et al. Trends and disparities in the utilization of thymectomy for myasthenia gravis in the United States. Neurology Clinical Practice. 2024;**14**(5):e200335

[58] Kesner VG, Oh SJ, Dimachkie MM, Barohn RJ. Lambert-Eaton myasthenic syndrome. Neurologic Clinics. 2018;**36**(2):379-394

[59] Titulaer MJ, Lang B, Verschuuren JJ. Lambert-Eaton myasthenic syndrome: From clinical characteristics to therapeutic strategies. Lancet Neurology. 2011;**10**(12):1098-1107

[60] Yoshikawa H, Adachi Y, Nakamura Y, Kuriyama N, Murai H, Nomura Y, et al. Nationwide survey of Lambert-Eaton myasthenic syndrome in Japan. BMJ Neurology Open. 2022;**4**(2):e000291

[61] Wirtz PW, Smallegange TM, Wintzen AR, Verschuuren JJ. Differences in clinical features between the Lambert-Eaton myasthenic syndrome with and without cancer: An analysis of 227 published cases. Clinical Neurology and Neurosurgery. 2002;**104**(4):359-363

[62] Wang Y, Xu C, Wang Y, Feng F, Wang H, Zhang Y, et al. Lambert-Eaton myasthenic syndrome in lung cancer. Contrast Media & Molecular Imaging. 2022;**2022**:3912376

[63] Lipka AF, Boldingh MI, van Zwet EW, Schreurs MWJ, Kuks JBM, Tallaksen CM, et al. Long-term follow-up, quality of life, and survival of patients with Lambert-Eaton myasthenic syndrome. Neurology. 2020;**94**(5):e511-e520

[64] Giannoccaro MP, Avoni P, Liguori R. Presynaptic paraneoplastic disorders of the neuromuscular junction: An update. Brain Sciences. 2021;**11**(8):1035

[65] Oh SJ, Kurokawa K, Claussen GC, Ryan HF. Electrophysiological diagnostic criteria of Lambert-Eaton myasthenic syndrome. Muscle & Nerve. 2005;**32**(4):515-520

[66] Meriney SD, Tarr TB, Ojala KS, Wu M, Li Y, Lacomis D, et al. Lambert-Eaton myasthenic syndrome: Mouse passive-transfer model illuminates disease pathology and facilitates testing therapeutic leads. Annals of the New York Academy of Sciences. 2018;**1412**(1):73-81

[67] Waterman SA. Voltage-gated calcium channels in autonomic neuroeffector transmission. Progress in Neurobiology. 2000;**60**(2):181-210

[68] Kimpinski K, Iodice V, Vernino S, Sandroni P, Low PA. Association of N-type calcium channel autoimmunity in patients with autoimmune autonomic ganglionopathy. Autonomic Neuroscience. 2009;**150**(1-2):136-139

[69] Rogers RS, Nishimune H. The role of laminins in the organization and function of neuromuscular junctions. Matrix Biology. 2017;**57-58**:86-105

[70] O'Neill JH, Murray NM, Newsom-Davis J. The Lambert-Eaton myasthenic syndrome. A review of 50 cases. Brain. 1988;**111**(Pt 3):577-596

[71] Smith RG, Appel SH. The Lambert-Eaton syndrome. Hospital Practice (Office Ed.). 1992;**27**(12):101-106, 111-3, 116

[72] Titulaer MJ, Wirtz PW, Kuks JBM, Schelhaas HJ, van der Kooi AJ, Faber CG, et al. The Lambert-Eaton myasthenic syndrome 1988-2008: A clinical picture in 97 patients. Journal of Neuroimmunology. 2008;**201-202**:153-158

[73] Poh M, Ming YC, Yanni PC, Ng GJ, Ho YH, Prasad K, et al. Postexercise reflex facilitation in Lambert-Eaton myasthenic syndrome. Practical Neurology. 2024;**24**(4):338-341

[74] Pellkofer HL, Voltz R, Kuempfel T. Favorable response to rituximab in a patient with anti-VGCC-positive Lambert-Eaton myasthenic syndrome and cerebellar dysfunction. Muscle & Nerve. 2009;**40**(2):305-308

[75] Bodkin C, Pascuzzi RM. Update in the management of myasthenia gravis and Lambert-Eaton myasthenic syndrome. Neurologic Clinics. 2021;**39**:133-146

Chapter 5

Vertigo in the Elderly

Firdevs Ezgi Uçan Tokuç

Abstract

Vertigo is a common symptom and a common cause of hospital admissions in the elderly. It can cause fractures in the elderly, especially due to falls, and contributes strongly to the burden of disability in people over 65 years of age. There are multiple etiologic causes of vertigo attacks in the elderly. This chapter will discuss the causes, symptoms, examination findings, and treatment modalities of vertigo in the elderly.

Keywords: central vertigo, peripheral vertigo, elderly, nystagmus, etiology

1. Introduction

Vertigo is a movement illusion defined as dizziness and a feeling of imbalance that may be observed as a result of peripheral or central pathologies [1]. Vertigo is one of the most common causes of neurological outpatient admissions. According to large population-based studies, 15–20% of adults are affected by vertigo every year [2]. This rate increases with age, and it has been reported that 34% of people over the age of 60 and 50% of people over the age of 85 are affected by vertigo [3].

Vertigo is a strong predictor of falls in the elderly. Skeletal muscle strength and mass decrease with aging, and the risk of injury due to falls increases in elderly patients. The mortality and morbidity of bone fractures, especially hip fractures, are quite high in these patients. Therefore, vertigo is becoming one of the strongest contributors to the burden of disability in people over the age of 65 [4]. There are multiple etiologic causes of vertigo episodes in the elderly. In addition to peripheral and central causes, psychiatric disorders, cardiovascular causes, and metabolic disorders may also cause vertigo, and a multidisciplinary approach is required. The etiology of vertigo in elderly age [5].

2. Differential diagnosis of peripheral vertigo and central vertigo

It is important to differentiate between peripheral and central vertigo as quickly as possible in patients presenting with vertigo due to differences in their etiology, pathogenesis, and treatment regimen. The assessment of patients should begin with a detailed anamnesis. The character and severity of dizziness; the presence and severity of nausea and vomiting; the presence, severity, and side of imbalance; and the presence of additional complaints such as hearing loss, pain in the ear, and tinnitus should be asked.

	Central	Peripheral
Nausea	Mild or none	Severe
Worsening with head movement	No	Yes
Oscillopsia	Severe	Mild
Imbalance	Severe	Mild to moderate
Hearing loss, tinnitus	Rare	Common
Abnormal neurological examination	Common	Rare
Recovery	Months or longer	Days or weeks
Latency after maneuver	Short (up to 5 seconds)	Long (up to 20 seconds)

Table 1.
Differential diagnosis of central and peripheral vertigo.

The differential diagnosis of peripheral vertigo and central vertigo is summarized in **Table 1** [6].

During follow-up, neuro-ophthalmological, neuro-otological, and neurological examinations of the patients should be performed completely. Eye movements should be evaluated, if nystagmus is observed, the direction of nystagmus/whether it changes with eye movements, the size of the pupils, the presence of direct/indirect light reflex must be tested.

HINTS (head impulse, nystagmus, test of skew) is one of the best clinical battery tests for the differential diagnosis of central and peripheral vertigo. The findings of the test are evaluated using the abbreviation INFARCT (impulse normal, fast-phase alternating, refixation on cover test) and help diagnose central vertigo. Head impulse test is performed by fixing the patient's eyes on an object and turning the patient's head rapidly to the right and left by 20 degrees and bringing it to the central position. The normal response is to keep the eyes on the target. If the eyes move with the head followed by a rapid corrective saccade, the test is positive and indicates a problem with the ipsilateral vestibulocochlear nerve, i.e., the problem is peripheral rather than central. Nystagmus: The presence of fast-phase alternating nystagmus or vertical nystagmus supports the diagnosis of unidirectional nystagmus peripheral vertigo, which suggests the diagnosis of central vertigo (**Table 2**). Test of skew: The patient's eyes are fixed on an object, and the eyes are closed one by one in turn. In the meantime, any vertical/diagonal corrective movement is observed (Refixation on Cover Test). Any abnormal movement supports central vertigo [7–11].

As a result, severe balance disorders, additional neurological symptoms and findings, and nystagmus with central features are in the foreground, and nausea is in the background in dizziness with central cause [9].

3. Central vertigo in the elderly

Central vertigo is a type of vertigo that develops as a result of dysfunction of the vestibular structures in the central nervous system. Neuroepithelial hair cells in the peripheral system consisting of saccule, utricle, and semicircular canals send projections to the vestibular nuclei in the caudal pons and rostral dorsolateral medulla via cranial nerve VIII (vestibulocochlear nerve). The vestibular nuclei on both sides are divided into four subnuclei: the superior vestibular nucleus, the lateral vestibular

	Central	Peripheral
Appearance	Vertical-horizontal/rotatory	Horizontal/rotatory
Latency	No latency	3–40 seconds
Change of direction	Varies with head position	Unidirectional (contralesional)
Fatigability	No	Yes
Effect of Fixation	No effect or may increase	Suppression
Dixx Hillpike Test	Sudden onset	Latent period

Table 2.
Differences between central and peripheral nystagmus.

nucleus, the medial vestibular nucleus, and the descending vestibular nucleus. These nuclei also receive afferent fibres from the cerebellum, reticular formation, spinal cord, and contralateral vestibular nucleus. Projections from the vestibular nuclei also extend to the cerebellum, extraocular nuclei, and spinal cord [7]. Therefore, any lesion observed in these localizations will result in central vertigo.

3.1 Etiology

Central vertigo in the elderly can be caused by many causes, such as ischaemia, infection, tumour and migraine, which can affect any area including the brain stem, spinal cord, and cerebellum from the eighth CN mentioned above (**Table 3**) [6].

In the following sections, central nervous system (CNS) diseases that can cause lesions resulting in central vertigo in the elderly will be discussed.

3.1.1 Cerebrovascular disease

3.1.1.1 Ischemic stroke

The vertebrobasilar system begins with the vertebral arteries arising from both subclavian arteries. Both vertebral arteries enter the cranium through the foramen

Causes of central vertigo
1. Cerebrovascular disease
2. Vestibular migraine
3. Multiple sclerosis
4. Central positional vertigo
5. Epilepsy
6. Craniocervical junction disorders
7. Tumors of the cerebellopontine angle and posterior fossa
8. Pareneoplastic cerebellar degeneration
9. Hereditary ataxia
10. The Others: Mal de debarquement syndrome, orthostatic hypotension, toxic (alcohol, drugs etc.), neurodegenerative disorders, infections (serebellitis) etc.

Table 3.
Causes of central vertigo.

magnum. At the level of the bulbus, it gives its largest branch, the posterior inferior cerebellar artery (PICA). At the level of the lower edge of the pons, both vertebral arteries merge to form the basilar artery. The basilar artery gives important branches such as the anterior inferior cerebellar artery (AICA) and superior cerebellar artery, which feed the cerebellum, pons, and mesencephalon and then terminates as the posterior cerebral artery [12]. Therefore, any ischaemic or haemorrhagic cerebrovascular event in the vertebrobasilar system will cause central vertigo. It is the most common and the most important and potentially life-threatening cause of central vertigo in the elderly. The diagnosis is made by cranial MRI.

3.1.1.1.1 PICA infarcts

PICA supplies the dorsolateral medulla where the vestibular nucleus complex is located, as well as the posterior inferior part of the cerebellum, cerebellar peduncle, and cerebellar tonsil. Lateral medullary syndrome (Wallenberg Syndrome) is the most common finding due to PICA infarcts. Dysphagia, dysarthria (nucleus ambiguus involvement), ipsilateral anhidrosis, miosis, ptosis (Horner's syndrome-involvement of sympathetic fibres), lack of pain and temperature sensation in the ipsilateral facial, (nucleus trigeminus involvement), ipsilateral cerebellar findings, lack of contralateral pain and temperature sensation (spinothalamic tract involvement), nausea, vomiting, vertigo, and nystagmus (involvement of the vestibular nucleus and pathways) are observed [13].

3.1.1.1.2 AICA infarcts

AICA supplies the middle and lower pons and part of the cerebellum. In the classical AICA syndrome that occurs due to ischaemia, vertigo, hearing loss, ipsilateral peripheral facial paralysis, ipsilateral Horner's syndrome, ipsilateral facial, contralateral arm, and leg hypoalgesia, ipsilateral ataxia, and nystagmus are observed [14].

3.1.1.1.3 Superior cerebellar artery infarcts

The superior cerebellar artery supplies the superior surface of the cerebellar hemisphere, the superior and middle cerebellar peduncles, and the pons. In superior cerebellar artery infarction, ataxia, nystagmus, and dysarthria are observed in addition to vertigo and vomiting, although less frequently compared to AICA and PICA infarctions [15].

3.1.1.2 Haemorrhagic stroke

Uncontrolled hypertension, amoloid angiopathy aneurysm, or AVM are common causes of hemorrhagic stroke in the elderly. Localized haemorrhages in the brain stem and cerebellum may cause acute vertigo, nausea, vomiting, and headaches. Progression may be rapid in massive cerebellar haematomas, and since acute hydrocephalus may develop due to compression of the fourth ventricle, diagnosis, treatment, and close clinical follow-up are of vital importance [13].

3.1.2 Vestibular migraine

Migraine and vertigo are common disorders in the general population and may coexist coincidentally. However, apart from these clinics, vertigo caused by migraine is called vestibular migraine and is observed in around 1% of the general population. Although it is usually seen in middle age, it can rarely be observed in the elderly, but the severity of the vertigo attack was higher in the elderly. Diagnostic criteria in the ICD-3 beta version are presented in **Table 4** [16, 17].

The temporal relationship between vertigo and migraine pain is variable, and positional or spontaneous vertigo attacks with a duration ranging from minutes to days are observed. Hearing loss and tinnitus are observed rarely and if present, they are mild and transient [16, 17].

3.1.3 Central positional vertigo

Central positional vertigo (CPV) shares common symptoms with benign paroxysmal positional vertigo (BPPV) and may be difficult to differentiate. Although BPPV is associated with "displaced otoconia in the semicircular canals," CPV results from impaired "central vestibular processing of canal and otolith activation, in addition, to prolonged velocity storage in the cerebellar nodulus" . In conclusion, it can develop as a result of any CNS lesion in the fourth ventricle, dorsal vertex, and vestibular nucleus.

Similar to BPPV, CPV is triggered by the position. However, it differs from BPVV especially with ophthalmological findings. Patients with BPVV have a short latency period after a provocative maneuver such as the Dix-Hallpike test. In CPV, vertigo has no latency period, and nystagmus starts immediately after positioning. The nystagmus in BPPV fatigues after some time in the head-hanging position, whereas the nystagmus in CPV may persist and is evident even after repetition of the position [18].

Vestibuler migraine
A. At least five attacks of moderate or severe vestibular symptoms lasting between 5 minutes and 72 hours
B. Recognized diagnosis of migraine
C. One or more of the following in at least 50% of vestibular attacks:
1. Headache with at least two of the following features
a. Unilateral location
b. Pulsatile
c. Moderate or severe intensity
d. Aggravation by physical activity
2. Photophobia and phonophobia
3. Visual aura
D. No other reasons to explain the dizziness
Probable vestibuler migraine
A. At least five attacks of moderate or severe vestibular symptoms lasting between 5 minutes and 72 hours
B. Presence of only one of the criteria B and C required for a final diagnosis
C. No other reason to explain the dizziness

Table 4.
Diagnostic criteria for vestibular migraine.

Features	CPV	BPPV
Latency	None	3–30 s
Duration of nystagmus	>30 s	<30 s
Persistent downbeat nystagmus	Yes	No
Nausea	+	+++
Worse with head movement	Yes	No
Evoked by Dix-Hallpike	+	+++
Resolves after maneuvers	No	Yes

BPVV: benign paroxysmal positional vertigo; CPV: central positional vertigo.

Table 5.
Features distinguishing CPV from BPPV.

In CPV, persistent downbeat nystagmus can be observed in any position (**Table 5**).

3.1.4 Epilepsy

Although vertigo due to epilepsy is rare, vertiginous epilepsy may occur owing to pre-seizure aura or side effects of some anti-seizure drugs including carbamazepine, phenyton, and oxcarbamezepine [19]. Video monitoring of blood drug levels helps in the diagnosis.

3.1.5 Craniocervical junction anomalies

In craniocervical junction abnormalities, spontal and positional vertigo, tinnitus, hearing loss, dysphonia, dysarthria, and sometimes hydrocephalus may be observed. Symptoms worsen with coughing and neck extension. Congenital fusion of the atlas and foremen magnum, atlantoaxial dislocation, platybasia and basilar invagination, and Chiari type-1 malformation may be observed [6].

3.1.6 Tumors of the cerebellopontine angle and posterior fossa

Acoustic neurinoma (vestibular schwannoma), the most common tumour of the cerebellopontine junction, is a benign tumour of the vestibular nerve. Progressive unilateral hearing loss, tinnitus, and ataxia are common. Cerebellopontine menenioma is the second most common tumour of the posterior fossa. Also, cerebellar tumours such as astrocytoma, ependymoma, and medulloblastoma cause central vertigo. Besides additional neurological symptoms, headaches are common in these patients [20].

3.1.7 Pareneoplastic cerebellar degeneration

Paraneoplastic neurological syndromes are antibody-associated inflammatory autoimmune neurological disorders not related to tumour metastasis or vascular or metabolic conditions. In paraneoplastic cerebellar degeneration, antibodies typically target the vestibulocerebellar tract, vestibular nucleus, and especially Purkinje cells.

It is particularly associated with ovarian, lung, and breast cancer, as well as Hodgkin's lymphoma. Some antibodies, such as Anti-Yo (breast and ovarian cancer),

Anti-Hu (small cell lung cancer), Anti-Ri (breast and ovarian cancer), Anti-TR and anti-mGluR1 (Hodgkin lymphoma), Anti-VGCC (small cell lung cancer), and Anti-Ma2 (small cell lung and testicular cancer), have been identified [21].

Cerebellar syndrome findings including rapidly progressive dizziness, vomiting, ataxia, dysarthria, and nystagmus as well as ophthalmoplegia and opsoclonus may be observed in patients [22].

It is important to consider the diagnosis, perform a lumbar puncture, and run antibody tests on both the body and itself. Cranial MRI is usually normal, and sometimes cerebellar atrophy may be observed. Malignancy screening should be performed if paraneoplastic cerebellar degeneration is diagnosed in patients without a diagnosis of malignancy. The prognosis is generally poor, rapid progression is observed within 6 months, and patients may become bedridden [22].

3.1.8 The other causes of central vertigo

3.1.8.1 Mal de debarquement syndrome

Mal de debarquement syndrome, which is defined as the perception of self-motion and instability following a passive movement, is usually seen after water travel, but also after air or land travel [23]. Although it can be seen at any age, it is more common in women over 50 years of age. The duration of symptoms usually ranges from a few minutes to a few hours, although there are rare cases with persistent symptoms lasting weeks and years [24, 25]. Patients are often unable to describe their feelings. They are typically described as "rocking," "swaying," or "swaying" or in phrases such as "I still feel like I am on a boat" or "it feels like I am walking on uneven ground," and anxiety and depression are common in these patients [23, 24]. Neurologic and physical examinations of the patients are normal, and cranial MRI and inner ear function test are normal [26].

3.1.8.2 Orthostatic hypotension

Orthostatic hypotension is common in the elderly. Symptoms of orthostatic hypotension can range from dizziness when first standing up to blackouts, sweating, nausea, and near-syncope/syncope. The most common causes are antihypertensive therapies, diseases causing autonomic neuropathy, and prolonged bed rest. It is diagnosed by the presence of a decrease of at least 20 mm Hg in systolic blood pressure or at least 10 mm Hg in diastolic blood pressure in a blood pressure measurement performed 3 minutes after changing from lying to standing position [27].

3.1.8.3 Drugs

Vertigo due to drug side effects is quite common, and many drugs can cause vertigo and dizziness. Due to age-related changes, multiple diseases, and polypharmacy, drug side effects and toxicities may be observed at lower doses and more frequently in the elderly. It includes anti-seizure medications (phenytoin, carbamazepine, lacosamide, oxcarbazepine, and lamotrigine), antidepressants (mirtazapine, sertraline, amitriptyline, and paroxetine), antihypertensive drugs (ACE inhibitors and calcium channel blockers), antibiotics (macrolides, ciprofloxacin, and aminoglycosides), and parkinsonian drugs (levodopa) [27].

4. Peripheral vertigo in the elderly

The most common cause of vertigo in the elderly is peripheral causes. In a review of 2148 elderly vertigo patients, the most common cause of vertigo was audio-vestibular diseases (AV) (28.4%). Among AV disorders, benign paroxysmal positional vertigo (BPPV) was the most common [28].

In this section, the main causes of peripheral vertigo in the elderly will be discussed.

4.1 Benign paroxysmal positional vertigo

Benign paroxysmal positional vertigo is characterized by transient vertigo and nystagmus caused by changes in the head position. It is the most common cause of peripheral vertigo and can occur at any age but is more common in the elderly [29].

Two main theories have been advocated in pathophysiology. Shuknecht argued that BPPV occurs when basophilic deposits adhere to the cupula in the posterior semicircular canal and called this pathologic finding "cupulolithiasis." Accordingly, the cupula becomes sensitive to gravity by the adhesion of otoconia to the cupula. When the head takes a hanging position, pathologic vestibuloocular reflex develops. With head movements, the cupula is displaced, resulting in vertigo and nystagmus due to endolymph movement [30, 31].

The latent period before the onset of nystagmus can be explained as the time for the displacement of the autoconia. The fatigability of nystagmus is explained by the dissolution of the otoconia in the endolymph [31].

Another theory is the 'canalilithiasis' theory advocated by Hall et al. Autochonia detached from the utricular macula move in the semicircular canal according to gravity and stimulate the endolymph duct cupula that they move with them. This results in the formation of a stimulation in the hair cells and vertigo and nystagmus [32].

Consequently, both theories are based on the displacement of autoconia. This is the reason why BPPV is more common in the elderly. Because the number and volume of otoliths decrease with age, and the connecting fibers between otoliths weaken. As a result, the otoconia detaches from the otolithic membrane and moves in the endolymph [31].

The diagnosis is made by anamnesis and provocation tests (Dix-Hallpike test). In the Dix-Hallpike Test, the patient is quickly moved from a sitting position to a lying position and the head is turned 45 degrees to the side by hanging 30 degrees lower than the horizontal plane. If vertigo and nystagmus are observed, the test is positive. Severe nausea may occur. However, caution is required, especially in elderly patients. The risk of dissection and stroke should be considered. Nystagmus in BPPV has distinctive features from central nystagmus: horizontoratory type, latent period, and fatigable nystagmus. The characteristics of nystagmus in BPPV are summarized in **Table 2**.

4.2 Meniere's disease

Recurrent episodes of vertigo lasting several hours with nausea and vomiting are typical in Meniere's Disease. Accompanying fluctuating hearing loss, a feeling of fullness in the ear and ringing in the ear are common. Meniere's disease is usually seen between the ages of 20 and 60, but it can be observed in 10–15% of patients over the age of 65. The pathophysiology is characterized by an increase in endolymph due to impaired absorption or release of endolymph and secondary membranous labyrinth dysfunction. The diagnosis includes anamnesis, otoscopic examination, and hearing test. Sensorimotor hearing loss at low frequencies is a typical finding for Meneiere's disease [33–35].

4.3 Vestibular neuritis

It is a sudden onset vertigo due to acute inflammation of the vestibular nerve and usually lasts longer than 24 hours. It is not accompanied by additional complaints such as hearing loss, ringing, and fullness in the ear. It is often preceded by a history of upper respiratory tract infection within a few weeks. Although it is usually seen between the ages of 30 and 60, recent studies have reported that it is common in individuals over the age of 70. Permanent dizziness develops in 30–40% of patients [36].

5. Treatment

Treatment of vertigo is especially important in the elderly to prevent falls and to prevent metabolic disorders that may occur due to vomiting. Medical treatment should consist of two steps. The first is symptomatic treatment with medication to relieve dizziness and vomiting. The second step is the treatment of the disease causing the vertigo.

In symptomatic treatments, drugs that are also used in the treatment of peripheral vertigo may be used: antihistamines (dimenhydrate, diphenhydramine, and meclizine), anticholinergic agents (scopolamine), benzodiazepines (diazepam and lorazepam), antiemetics (metoclopramide), betahistidine, and piracetam [37–39].

The second step of treatment depends on the underlying cause. If the cause of vertigo is acute ischemic stroke, IV thrombolytic therapies and/or endovascular therapies can be used in appropriate patients with promising results. Antiplatelet agents should be used in noncardioembolic stroke, and anticoagulant agents should be used in cardioembolic stroke [40]. In hemorrhagic stroke, blood pressure should be controlled, and reabsorption of bleeding should be expected.

Treatment of vestibular migraine is similar to the treatment of migraine acute attacks and may include prophylaxis and symptomatic treatment for vertigo. Prophylactic treatment may include beta-blockers as well as antiseizure medications such as topiramate or valproic acid [41]. In a prospective multicenter study of metoprolol in prophylactic treatment to reduce the frequency of attacks, metoprolol was not superior to placebo [42]. IV immunoglobulin, corticosteroids, or plasma exchange are treatment options for paraneoplastic cerebellar degeneration. In mal de debarquement syndrome, treatment options are limited, and benzodiazepines may show benefit. Most commonly, clonazepam 0.25–0.5 mg twice daily is used [24]. In addition to medical treatment, balance, posture and eye stabilization, physical exercises, and physiotherapies should be among the supportive treatments [43].

In addition to drug therapies, Epley maneuver, which is a repositioning maneuver, gives very good results in the treatment of BPPV. The aim of the maneuver is to move the canaliculi at appropriate angles in the posterior semicircular canal so that they fall into the utricus. The person performing the test stands behind the patient. The patient is first turned 45 degrees towards the unaffected ear in a sitting position and then placed on the back, and the head is supported with the hands and brought to extension. The head is then turned at a 45-degree angle towards the intact ear without breaking the extension. Then, the body and head are turned together by 90 degrees more than in the supine position, and the head is turned 135 degrees to the vertical plane. Finally, the patient is placed in a sitting position, and the head is tilted 20–30 degrees forward. While performing this maneuver, the head should wait in each position until the latent period and nystagmus end [44].

6. Conclusion

Vertigo is a common complaint in the elderly. Clinical history and detailed neuro-otologic examinations are essential to evaluate vertigo in the elderly population. Neurologic examination and Dix-Hallpike test should be performed in the elderly, as peripheral causes as well as central causes such as stroke, which require urgent treatment, are involved in the etiology. In addition to symptomatic drug treatments, there are etiologic treatments.

Conflict of interest

The authors declare no conflict of interest.

Author details

Firdevs Ezgi Uçan Tokuç
Antalya Provincal Health Directorate Antalya Training and Research Hospital, Antalya, Türkiye

*Address all correspondence to: ezgiucan@gmail.com

References

[1] Akdal G. Vertigo ve Dengesizlik. In: Öğe EA, Baykan B, Bilgiç B, editors. ITF Nöroloji. 4th ed. Nöbel Tıp Kitapevi; 2021. pp. 493-500

[2] Neuhauser HK. The epidemiology of dizziness and vertigo. Handbook of Clinical Neurology. 2016;**137**:67-82. DOI: 10.1016/B978-0-444-63437-5.00005-4

[3] Jönsson R, Sixt E, Landahl S, Rosenhall U. Prevalence of dizziness and vertigo in an urban elderly population. Journal of Vestibular Research. 2004;**14**(1):47-52

[4] Fernández L, Breinbauer HA, Delano PH. Vertigo and dizziness in the elderly. Frontiers in Neurology. 2015;**6**:144. Published 2015 Jun 26. DOI: 10.3389/fneur.2015.00144

[5] Swain SK, Anand N, Mishra S. Vertigo among elderly people: Current opinion. Journal of Medical Society. 2019;**33**:1-5

[6] Karatas M. Central vertigo and dizziness: Epidemiology, differential diagnosis, and common causes. The Neurologist. 2008;**14**(6):355-364

[7] Lui F, Foris LA, Willner K, et al. Central vertigo. In: StatPearls. Treasure Island (FL): StatPearls Publishing; 2024. Available from: https://www.ncbi.nlm.nih.gov/books/NBK441861/

[8] Von Martial R, Leinweber C, Hubert N, et al. Feasibility of telemedical HINTS (head impulse-nystagmus-test of skew) evaluation in patients with acute dizziness or vertigo in the emergency department of primary care hospitals. Frontiers in Neurology. 2022;**12**:768460. DOI: 10.3389/fneur.2021.768460

[9] Kerber KA. Acute constant dizziness. CONTINUUM Lifelong Learning in Neurology. 2012;**18**(5):1041-1059

[10] Kerber KA, Baloh RW. The evaluation of a patient with dizziness. Neurology: Clinical Practise. 2011;**1**(1):24-33. DOI: 10.1212/CPJ.0b013e31823d07b6

[11] Strupp M, Brandt T. Central vertigo. An International Journal of Otorhinolaryngology Clinics. 2012;**4**(2):71-76. DOI: 10.5005/jp-journals-10003-1089

[12] Piccinin MA, Munakomi S. Neuroanatomy, vertebrobasilar system. In: StatPearls. Treasure Island (FL): StatPearls Publishing; 2024. Available from: https://www.ncbi.nlm.nih.gov/books/NBK540995/

[13] Chakor RT, Eklare N. Vertigo in Cerebrovascular diseases. An International Journal of Otorhinolaryngology Clinics. 2012;**4**(1):46-53. DOI: 10.5005/jp-journals-10003-1087

[14] İlhan Algın D, Korkmaz D, Yalın Ş. Bilateral anterior inferior serebellar arter infarktı. Turkish Journal of Cerebrovascular Diseases. 2012;**18**(1):20-22. DOI: 10.5505/tbdhd.2012.02996

[15] Ioannides K, Tadi P, Naqvi IA. Cerebellar infarct. In: StatPearls. Treasure Island (FL): StatPearls Publishing; 2024. Available from: https://www.ncbi.nlm.nih.gov/books/NBK470416/

[16] International Headache Society. The International Classification of Headache Disorders, 3rd edition (beta version). Cephalalgia. 2013;**33**(9):629-808

[17] Stolte B, Holle D, Naegel S, et al. Vestibular migraine. Cephalalgia. 2015;**35**(3):262-270. DOI: 10.1177/0333102414535113

[18] De Schutter E, Adham ZO, Kattah JC. Central positional vertigo: A clinical-imaging study. Progress in Brain Research. 2019;**249**:345-360. DOI: 10.1016/bs.pbr.2019.04.022

[19] Tarnutzer AA, Lee SH, Robinson KA, et al. Clinical and electrographic findings in epileptic vertigo and dizziness: A systematic review. Neurology. 2015;**84**(15):1595-1604. DOI: 10.1212/WNL.0000000000001474

[20] Halmagyi MG, Akdal G. Vertigo and imbalance. Journal of Neurological Sciences (Turkish). 2005;**22**(2):123-141

[21] Aly R, Emmady PD. Paraneoplastic cerebellar degeneration. In: StatPearls. Treasure Island (FL): StatPearls Publishing; 2024. Available from: https://www.ncbi.nlm.nih.gov/books/NBK560638/

[22] Loehrer PA, Zieger L, Simon OJ. Update on paraneoplastic cerebellar degeneration. Brain Sciences. 2021;**11**(11):1414. DOI: 10.3390/brainsci11111414

[23] Ombergen AV, Rompaey VV, Maes LK, et al. Mal de debarquement syndrome: A systematic review. Journal of Neurology. 2016;**263**(5):843-854. DOI: 10.1007/s00415-015-7962-6

[24] Cha YH. Mal de debarquement. Seminars in Neurology. 2009;**29**:520-527. DOI: 10.1055/s-0029-1241038

[25] Mucci V, Canceri JM, Brown R, et al. Mal de debarquement Syndrome: A survey on subtypes, misdiagnoses, onset and associated psychological features. Journal of Neurology. 2018;**265**:486-499. DOI: 10.1007/s00415-017-8725-3

[26] Brown J, Baloh R. Persistent mal de debarquement syndrome: A motion-induced subjective disorder of balance. American Journal of Otolaryngology. 1987;**8**(4):219-222. DOI: 10.1016/s0196-0709(87)80007-8

[27] Gnerre P, Casati C, Frualdo M, et al. Management of vertigo: From evidence to clinical practice. Italian Journal of Medicine. 2015;**9**:180-192. DOI: 10.4081/itjm.2015.437

[28] Fancello V, Hatzopoulos S, Santopietro G, Fancello G, Palma S, Skarżyński PH, et al. Vertigo in the elderly: A systematic literature review. Journal of Clinical Medicine. 2023;**12**(6):2182. DOI: 10.3390/jcm12062182

[29] Neuhauser HK, von Brevern M, Radtke A, Lezius F, Feldmann M, Ziese T, et al. Epidemiology of vestibular vertigo: A neurotologic survey of the general population. Neurology. 2005;**65**(6):898-904. DOI: 10.1212/01.wnl.0000175987.59991.3d. Erratum in: Neurology. 2006;67(8):1528

[30] Schuknecht HF. Cupulolithiasis. Archives of Otolaryngology. 1969;**90**(6):765-778. DOI: 10.1001/archotol.1969.00770030767020

[31] Balatsouras DG, Koukoutsis G, Fassolis A, Moukos A, Apris A. Benign paroxysmal positional vertigo in the elderly: Current insights. Clinical Interventions in Aging. 2018;**13**:2251-2266. Published 2018 Nov 5. DOI: 10.2147/CIA.S144134

[32] Hall SF, Ruby RR, McClure JA. The mechanics of benign paroxysmal vertigo. The Journal of Otolaryngology. 1979;**8**(2):151-158

[33] Vibert D, Caversaccio M, Häusler R. Meniere's disease in the elderly. Otolaryngologic Clinics of North America. 2010;**43**(5):1041-1046. DOI: 10.1016/j.otc.2010.05.009

[34] Ballester M, Liard P, Vibert D, Hausler R. Meniere's disease in the elderly. Otology & Neurotology. 2002;**23**(1):73-78. DOI: 10.1097/00129492-200201000-00017

[35] Bayındır T, Kalcıoğlu MT. Periferik Vertigo. Italian Journal of Medicine. 2010;**17**(2):155-163

[36] Bae CH, Na HG, Choi YS. Current diagnosis and treatment of vestibular neuritis: A narrative review. Journal of Yeungnam Medical Science. 2022;**39**(2):81-88. DOI: 10.12701/yujm.2021.01228

[37] Berisavac II, Pavlović AM, Trajković JJ, et al. Drug treatment of vertigo in neurological disorders. Neurology India. 2015;**63**(6):933-939. DOI: 10.4103/0028-3886.170097

[38] Arhami Dolatabadi A, Larimi SR, Safaie A. Oral piracetam vs betahistine in outpatient management of peripheral vertigo; a randomized clinical trial. Archives of Academic Emergency Medicine. 2019;7(1):e9

[39] Gekht AB, Vialkova AB, Galanov DV. Clinico-neurological and stabilometric analysis of betahistine (betaserc) efficacy in the patients with vertigo in the rehabilitation period of ischemic stroke. Zhurnal Nevrologii i Psikhiatrii Imeni S.S. Korsakova. 2005;(Suppl. 15):32-38

[40] Del Brutto VJ, Chaturvedi S, Diener HC, Romano JG, Sacco RL. Antithrombotic therapy to prevent recurrent strokes in ischemic cerebrovascular disease: JACC scientific expert panel. Journal of the American College of Cardiology. 2019;**74**(6):786-803. DOI: 10.1016/j.jacc.2019.06.039

[41] Strupp M, Dieterich M, Brandt T. The treatment and natural course of peripheral and central vertigo. Deutsches Ärzteblatt International. 2013;**110**(29-30):505-515; quiz 515-6. DOI: 10.3238/arztebl.2013.0505. Epub 2013 Jul 22

[42] Bayer O, Adrion C, Al Tawil A, Mansmann U, Strupp M, PROVEMIG investigators. Results and lessons learnt from a randomized controlled trial: Prophylactic treatment of vestibular migraine with metoprolol (PROVEMIG). Trials. 2019;**20**(1):813. Published 2019 Dec 30. DOI: 10.1186/s13063-019-3903-5

[43] Stephen CD, Brizzi KT, Bouffard MA, et al. The comprehensive management of cerebellar ataxia in adults. Current Treatment Options in Neurology. 2019;**21**(3):9. Published 2019 Feb 21. DOI: 10.1007/s11940-019-0549-2

[44] Dağkıran M, Sürmelioğlu Ö, Ay Ö. Benign Paroksismal Pozisyonel Vertigoda Tanı ve Tedavi Yöntemleri. Arşiv Kaynak Tarama Dergisi. 2015;**24**(4):555-564

Chapter 6

Chronic Pain in Elderly: Emerging Challenges and Updates about Line of Care and Pathways

Caroline Bozzetto Ambrosi and Patricia Bozzetto Ambrosi

Abstract

This chapter aims to provide the best guidance for academics and clinicians regarding the emerging challenges and updates about the line of care and pathways of chronic pain in the elderly. A comprehensive review of pain concepts and their consequences, as well as the latest evidence on biological and neurological pathways of chronic pain, then focusing on the care pathways in older adults, especially in its assessment and diagnosis, multimodal interventions and interdisciplinary care that links aging and pain, in addition to its challenges and barriers for the care pathway in older adults is also presented. Furthermore, ongoing research and innovations that are crucial to the advancement of chronic pain management in older adults will be discussed, offering new hope for more effective and safe treatments to improve the quality of life of older adults living with chronic pain.

Keywords: chronic disease, elderly, public health, rehabilitation, comprehensive health care, health care line

1. Introduction

Pain itself is associated with substantial disability due to reduced mobility, avoidance of activities, falls, depression and anxiety, sleep impairment and isolation. Its negative effects extend beyond the patient to disrupt family and social relationships. On the other hand, it is important to note that acute pain serves as a warning signal to the body, unlike chronic pain, which generally does not have a clear protective or beneficial function and specifically represents a significant economic burden for society [1–5].

In the elderly, chronic pain is a particularly relevant condition because it often coexists with multiple comorbidities, and it can be extremely challenging to manage due to the physiological changes associated with aging. These specific changes include altered pain perception, reduced pain tolerance and an increased sensitivity to pain due to nerve degeneration and changes in central nervous system processing. The main causes of chronic pain in the elderly to be highlighted are primarily secondary to another previous disorder, including cancer, neuropathic pain, musculoskeletal

 IntechOpen

disorders, chronic post-traumatic or post-surgical pain, chronic visceral pain, chronic headache and orofacial pain, among others [2, 4].

However, chronic pain is typically defined as "pain that lasts or recurs for more than 3–6 months" and is classified as primary (such as fibromyalgia)—when the pain is the disease itself—or secondary—when it is related to another previous disease (e.g., cancer-related pain) or beyond the expected healing period of an injury or disease. Then chronic pain is one of the most common conditions encountered in clinical practice, particularly among older patients (≥65 years) [3–5].

2. Prevalence and consequences of chronic pain in the elderly

The prevalence of chronic pain in older adults has significant consequences for their overall well-being and quality of life. The consequences include: (i) reduced mobility, as pain can limit physical activity, leading to muscle weakness, joint stiffness and an increased risk of falls; (ii) sleep disturbances: chronic pain often interferes with sleep, leading to fatigue and worsening other health problems; (iii) mental health problems: there is a strong association between chronic pain and depression, anxiety and cognitive decline in older adults; (iv) social isolation: pain can lead to withdrawal from social activities, resulting in loneliness and further decline in mental health [6, 7].

In older adults living in the community, chronic pain is commonly reported at approximately 50% of the frequency. The true prevalence may be higher due to underreporting, as many older adults consider pain a normal part of aging and may not report it or seek medical help [8]. Chronic pain is more commonly reported among older women than men, which may be attributed to the higher incidence of conditions such as osteoarthritis and osteoporosis in women, as well as possible differences in the perception and reporting of pain. This shows that there is a well-established gender difference [6–9].

Systematic studies have shown that the prevalence of low back pain among the elderly population ranged from 2/3 of the population studied and this pain condition led to functional disability in 60% of the studies. Studies with a lower frequency of objectively reported pain, however, were associated with poorer health perception, poorer quality of life and depressive symptoms [8–11].

According to Molton and Terril, an overview of persistent pain in the elderly showed the prevalence of low back pain due to osteoarthritis, especially in the lower back or neck (approximately 65%), musculoskeletal pain (approximately 40%), peripheral neuropathic pain (usually due to diabetes or postherpetic neuralgia—35%) and chronic joint pain (15–25%) [5]. Surprisingly, the estimated prevalence of chronic pain is higher, from 25% to 50% in community-dwelling elderly people, reaching 80% in institutionalized individuals [10].

In nursing home residents, the prevalence of chronic pain is typically higher in nursing homes, with studies showing that up to 80% of residents suffer from some form of chronic pain. This may be related to a higher burden of comorbidities and a higher prevalence of conditions such as dementia, which can complicate pain assessment and treatment [6–11].

Several other factors are responsible for the impact of comorbidities. It is quite clear that conditions such as diabetes, cardiovascular disease and obesity, which are more common in older adults, can exacerbate chronic pain. In addition, mental health issues such as depression and anxiety, which are also prevalent in older adults, can intensify the experience of pain. Other important factors reported in the literature that have been associated with this increase are obesity epidemics, with body mass index (BMI) being considered a risk factor for increased trends in mild to severe pain in both women and men [11, 12].

Other studies proposed that older age and at least one comorbidity were predictors of chronic musculoskeletal pain in older adults. An additional longitudinal cohort analysis, conducted in older individuals (>75 years), suggested that peripheral arterial disease, low back pain, high BMI and female gender are associated with a higher risk of experiencing pain in old age. At the same time, smoking cessation may be responsible for a reduction in pain syndromes in the elderly [1, 6–11].

Domenichiello and Ramsden [6], aging can be considered a risk factor for chronic pain, being a primary cause of disability or a consequence of other diseases commonly seen in geriatric patients. Persistent pain in the elderly has major impacts on health system costs due to the complexity of treatment and the exacerbation of psychological conditions, including anxiety, depression, insomnia and low levels of quality of life. Notably, the authors point out that long-lasting pain may represent a risk factor for mortality in the elderly, worsening common problems such as cognitive deficits and insufficient social interaction [6].

Additional studies on pain in the elderly will help to bridge the gaps in the prevalence and incidence of pain in this population. This is relevant to improve pain diagnosis and guide interdisciplinary teams in the treatment of these individuals, aiming to achieve global health benefits [13, 14].

3. Biological and neurological pathways

An aversion to the sensation of pain causes a person to avoid situations in which they will be exposed to physical harm. In acute pain, this mechanism can prevent the worsening of a recent injury. On the other hand, chronic pain can reduce a person's daily activities and limit social contacts, negatively influencing their quality of life, with harmful consequences for their health. In this process, there are three biological mechanisms involved in pain: nociceptive, neuropathic and nociplastic. These often coexist, which sometimes results in the term "mixed pain" [6–14].

Understanding the biological and neurological pathways that underlie chronic pain in the elderly is crucial for developing effective management strategies. Aging leads to significant changes in pain perception and processing, with neuropathic and inflammatory mechanisms playing key roles in the persistence of chronic pain. By addressing these underlying mechanisms as illustrated in the flow chart above, healthcare providers can better tailor interventions to alleviate chronic pain and improve the quality of life for elderly patients [15, 16].

3.1 Aging and pain sensitivity

Aging affects the body's pain sensitivity through several complex mechanisms involving both the peripheral and central nervous systems. Three important changes happen inherent to elderly age that will be discussed further. As people age, peripheral changes happen. There is a gradual loss of nerve fibers in the peripheral nervous system, leading to reduced sensitivity to pain stimuli (hypoalgesia) in some cases. However, this does not necessarily translate to reduced pain experience. Aging also causes structural and functional changes in the nociceptors (pain receptors) and a decrease in the speed of nerve conduction. These changes can alter the perception of pain, sometimes leading to paradoxical outcomes, such as an increased sensation of pain (hyperalgesia) due to an imbalance between excitatory and inhibitory signals in the nervous system [16, 17].

On the other side, the central nervous system, central changes and aging lead to alterations in pain processing pathways, including reduced plasticity of neurons and changes in neurotransmitter levels. This can result in changes in the way pain is processed and perceived. The brain regions responsible for processing pain signals, such as the thalamus and somatosensory cortex, may undergo atrophy, leading to altered pain perception. Moreover, the descending pain modulatory system, which normally helps suppress pain, may become less effective with age, contributing to increased pain sensitivity. Cognitive decline and emotional changes, such as increased anxiety or depression, can also affect pain perception. Cognitive and emotional Influences when older adults may experience pain more intensely due to these factors, as the brain's ability to filter out or cope with pain diminishes [15–17].

3.2 Neuropathic pain mechanisms

Neuropathic pain, a type of chronic pain resulting from damage to or dysfunction of the nervous system, is particularly relevant in the elderly due to age-related neurological changes. Central Sensitization: This refers to a condition where the central nervous system becomes hypersensitive to pain stimuli. Even mild stimuli that would not normally cause pain can become painful. Aging can exacerbate central sensitization due to changes in the spinal cord's dorsal horn and other central pain processing areas. This hypersensitivity is often linked to conditions like fibromyalgia and is more prevalent in older adults due to the cumulative impact of chronic pain and repeated activation of pain pathways. Neuroinflammation: Aging is associated with an increase in neuroinflammatory processes, where immune cells in the nervous system (like microglia and astrocytes) become activated and contribute to pain. This inflammation can enhance the perception of pain and sustain chronic pain states, making pain management more challenging. Peripheral Neuropathy: Peripheral neuropathy, a common cause of neuropathic pain in the elderly, often results from conditions like diabetes, chemotherapy or simply age-related degeneration of peripheral nerves. These damaged nerves can send abnormal pain signals to the brain even in the absence of an actual pain stimulus, leading to sensations such as burning, tingling or shooting pain [15–18].

3.3 Inflammatory pathways

Inflammation plays a critical role in chronic pain, particularly in conditions like arthritis, where inflammation of the joints leads to persistent pain. With aging, the inflammatory response undergoes significant changes that can exacerbate chronic pain [17, 18]. Inflammaging: This term describes the chronic, low-grade inflammation associated with aging. It results from the accumulation of proinflammatory cytokines (like IL-6, TNF-alpha and CRP) and the reduced efficacy of the body's anti-inflammatory mechanisms. This persistent inflammation can lead to the sensitization of pain pathways and contribute to the development and maintenance of chronic pain conditions, particularly in musculoskeletal disorders. Joint and Tissue Degeneration: In conditions like osteoarthritis, age-related wear and tear on joints can lead to the release of inflammatory mediators that sustain pain. The synovial

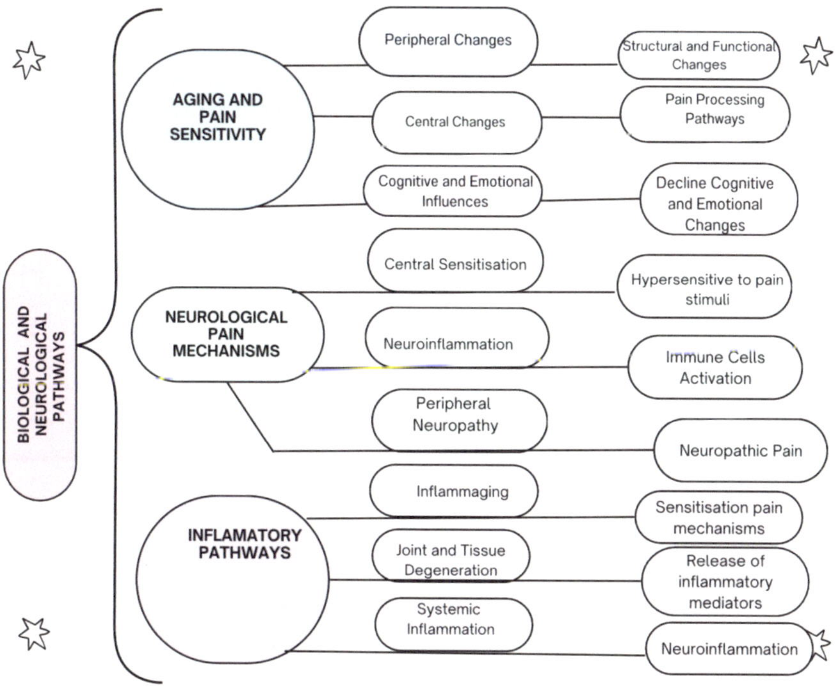

Figure 1.
Flowchart about biological and neurological mechanisms of chronic pain.

fluid, cartilage and other joint components undergo degeneration, leading to inflammation that perpetuates pain and limits mobility. Systemic Inflammation: Aging is associated with a general increase in systemic inflammation, which can exacerbate conditions like rheumatoid arthritis and contribute to other forms of chronic pain. This systemic inflammation can also affect the central nervous system, leading to neuroinflammation and contributing to the development of chronic pain syndromes (**Figure 1**) [19, 20].

4. Line of care and pathways in chronic pain management

Chronic pain management in the elderly requires a comprehensive, individualized approach that integrates pharmacological and non-pharmacological interventions, supported by an interdisciplinary care team. By addressing the unique challenges posed by aging, healthcare providers can improve pain management and overall well-being in older adults [21–23].

4.1 Assessment and diagnosis

4.1.1 Comprehensive pain assessment tools tailored for the elderly

Accurately assessing chronic pain in the elderly is crucial but challenging due to factors like cognitive decline, communication barriers and the presence of multiple comorbidities. Comprehensive pain assessment in elderly patients should be multidimensional, encompassing physical, emotional and functional aspects [21–26]. Before, outlining a treatment plan, a comprehensive pain assessment is essential for making a specific diagnosis and ensuring targeted therapy whenever possible.

When assessing chronic pain, a range of settings of clinical practice are essential to be shown:

i. *Pain assessment scales:* Tools like the numeric rating scale (NRS), visual analog scale (VAS) and verbal descriptor scale (VDS) are commonly used but may need adaptation for older adults with cognitive impairment. The Pain Assessment in Advanced Dementia (PAINAD) Scale is particularly useful for those who cannot verbally communicate their pain, as it relies on observations of behaviors like facial expressions, body language and vocalizations.

ii. *Multidimensional assessment tools*: The Brief Pain Inventory (BPI) and the McGill pain questionnaire provide a more comprehensive evaluation by assessing the intensity of pain, its impact on daily activities and the patient's emotional response to pain. The Geriatric Pain Measure (GPM) is specifically designed for older adults, covering various aspects of pain and its impact on physical and social functioning.

iii. *Functional assessment:* Evaluating how pain affects an elderly person's ability to perform activities of daily living (ADLs) is essential. Tools like the activities of daily living (ADL) scale and the instrumental activities of daily living (IADL) scale help in understanding the impact of pain on the patient's independence.

4.2 Differentiating between chronic pain and acute conditions

It is important to distinguish between chronic pain, which persists for long periods and often lacks a clear etiology, and acute pain, which is usually associated with injury or disease and has a well-defined onset. In the elderly, this distinction can be challenging because acute conditions like fractures or infections can exacerbate existing chronic pain or be misinterpreted as worsening chronic conditions. A thorough medical history and physical examination are critical. Clinicians should ask about the duration, location and character of the pain, and any recent changes that might suggest an acute condition superimposed on chronic pain. Imaging studies (e.g., X-rays and MRI) and laboratory tests can help identify acute pathologies, such as fractures, infections or malignancies, that might be contributing to or mimicking chronic pain [22, 27].

Various treatment options are available for chronic pain management in the elderly including either pharmacological or non-pharmacological interventions.

4.3 Pharmacological interventions overview of commonly used analgesics

- *Non-Steroidal Anti-Inflammatory Drugs (NSAIDs)*: NSAIDs are frequently used for conditions like osteoarthritis. However, they come with significant risks for the elderly, including gastrointestinal bleeding, cardiovascular events and renal impairment. The use of COX-2 inhibitors, which have a lower risk of gastrointestinal side effects, might be considered, but these also carry cardiovascular risks.

- *Opioids*: While opioids can be effective for managing moderate to severe pain, their use in the elderly must be approached with caution due to the risks of sedation, respiratory depression, constipation and the potential for dependency. Doses should be started low and titrated slowly, with close monitoring for side effects. Long-acting formulations are often preferred to avoid the peaks and troughs associated with short-acting opioids.

- *Acetaminophen (Paracetamol)*: Acetaminophen is considered safer for mild to moderate pain management in the elderly, particularly for musculoskeletal pain. However, care must be taken to avoid exceeding the recommended dose, as the risk of liver toxicity increases, especially in those with underlying liver conditions or those who consume alcohol [28, 29].

4.4 Emerging treatments

- *Neuromodulation*: Techniques like *spinal cord stimulation (SCS)* and *transcutaneous electrical nerve stimulation (TENS)* are increasingly used in elderly patients with chronic neuropathic pain. These therapies modulate pain signals through electrical impulses, offering pain relief with fewer systemic side effects compared to pharmacological treatments [30].

- *Biologics*: For conditions like rheumatoid arthritis, biological agents targeting specific inflammatory pathways (e.g., TNF inhibitors and IL-6 inhibitors) have become an important part of the treatment arsenal. These agents can provide significant pain relief by reducing underlying inflammation, though their use must be carefully monitored in the elderly due to the risk of infections and other side effects [20–29].

4.5 Non-pharmacological interventions physical therapy and exercise regimens

Physical therapy plays a vital role in managing chronic pain in the elderly, aiming to improve mobility, strength and overall function.

- *Tailored exercise programs*: Exercise regimens should be individualized based on the patient's physical capabilities and limitations. Low-impact activities like walking, swimming and yoga can be effective in reducing pain and improving function. Strength training and balance exercises are particularly important in reducing the risk of falls, which is a major concern in the elderly [31].

- *Manual therapy*: Techniques like massage, myofascial release and joint mobilization can provide relief from musculoskeletal pain. These therapies can help reduce muscle tension, improve circulation and enhance flexibility [32].

4.6 Psychological approaches

- *Cognitive behavioral therapy (CBT)*: CBT is one of the most effective psychological interventions for chronic pain, helping patients change the way they think about and respond to pain. It can reduce pain intensity, improve coping skills and enhance quality of life [33].

- *Mindfulness and relaxation techniques*: Mindfulness-based stress reduction (MBSR) and relaxation techniques like *deep breathing* and *progressive muscle relaxation* can help reduce the perception of pain and the emotional distress associated with it [32, 34].

4.7 Alternative therapies

- *Acupuncture*: Acupuncture is increasingly recognized as a complementary therapy for chronic pain. It may help by stimulating the release of endorphins and modulating pain pathways [35].

- *Chiropractic care*: For certain musculoskeletal pain conditions, chiropractic adjustments can provide relief by improving spinal alignment and function. However, this should be approached cautiously in the elderly due to the risk of injury [36].

- *Diet and supplements*: Dietary modifications and supplements like omega-3 fatty acids, glucosamine and turmeric may offer anti-inflammatory benefits and help manage pain, particularly in conditions like osteoarthritis. Adequate intake of vitamin D and calcium is also important for bone health [37].

4.8 Interdisciplinary care

4.8.1 Importance of a multidisciplinary approach

Effective chronic pain management in the elderly often requires a team-based approach involving multiple healthcare professionals.

- *Primary care physicians*: They often serve as the first point of contact and can coordinate care, ensuring that all aspects of the patient's health are addressed.

- *Pain specialists*: These professionals can provide more specialized care, including interventional procedures, advanced pharmacological management and guidance on emerging therapies.

- *Physical therapists*: They design and implement exercise and rehabilitation programs tailored to the patient's needs and physical abilities.

- *Mental health professionals*: Addressing the psychological components of chronic pain is crucial, particularly in elderly patients who may suffer from depression or anxiety. Psychologists or psychiatrists can offer CBT, medication management and other therapies to support mental well-being [33].

4.9 Coordinating care and communication

- *Interdisciplinary meetings*: Regular communication between team members is essential for developing and adjusting the care plan. Interdisciplinary meetings can help ensure that all aspects of the patient's pain are being addressed and that treatments are coordinated effectively [38].

- *Patient and family involvement*: Engaging the patient and their family in the care process is critical. Educating them about the nature of chronic pain, treatment options and the importance of adherence to the care plan can improve outcomes and enhance the patient's quality of life.

5. Challenges and barriers in line of care

Addressing the challenges and barriers in chronic pain management for the elderly requires a multifaceted approach. Underreporting and undertreatment of pain are major issues, often rooted in misconceptions, communication barriers and systemic limitations. Overcoming these challenges involves improving pain assessment, enhancing provider education, ensuring better access to care and empowering patients and their families through education. By addressing these barriers, healthcare providers can improve the quality of life for elderly patients suffering from chronic pain [22].

5.1 Underreporting and undertreatment

5.1.1 Why chronic pain in the elderly is often underreported?

Chronic pain in the elderly is frequently underreported due to several factors:

- *Perception of pain as a normal part of aging:* Many elderly individuals believe that pain is an inevitable part of aging and therefore do not report it to healthcare providers. This perception can be reinforced by societal attitudes and even by some healthcare providers, leading to a normalization of pain that discourages active reporting.

- *Communication barriers:* Cognitive decline, dementia and sensory impairments (e.g., hearing or vision loss) can make it difficult for elderly patients to effectively communicate their pain. Additionally, some older adults may have difficulty articulating the intensity or nature of their pain, particularly if they are experiencing complex or diffuse pain symptoms.

- *Fear of diagnosis and treatment:* Some elderly patients may avoid reporting pain due to fear of a serious diagnosis or the potential consequences of treatment, such as surgery or long-term medication use. Concerns about side effects, addiction (particularly with opioids) and the stigma associated with taking pain medications can also lead to underreporting.

- *Stoicism and cultural factors:* Cultural attitudes toward pain and aging can influence whether an elderly person reports pain. In some cultures, stoicism and enduring pain without complaint are valued, which can lead to underreporting. Gender differences can also play a role, with some studies suggesting that men may be less likely to report pain than women.

5.1.2 Why chronic pain is often undertreated?

- *Misdiagnosis or lack of recognition:* Chronic pain in the elderly is often undertreated because it may be misdiagnosed or not recognized as a significant health issue. Pain symptoms might be attributed to other chronic conditions or dismissed as a natural consequence of aging without proper investigation.

- *Complexity of pain management:* Managing chronic pain in the elderly is complicated by the presence of multiple comorbidities, which can make it difficult to prescribe effective treatments without risking adverse effects. Polypharmacy (the use of multiple medications) is common in this population, increasing the risk of drug interactions and side effects, which can lead to more conservative pain management approaches.

- *Inadequate pain assessment:* Even when pain is reported, it may not be adequately assessed. Healthcare providers may rely on standard pain scales that are not well-suited to elderly patients, particularly those with cognitive impairments. Inadequate assessment can lead to undertreatment, as the full extent of the pain may not be appreciated.

- *Provider attitudes and knowledge gaps:* Some healthcare providers may have limited training in pain management, particularly in geriatric populations. This can result in underprescribing of pain medications, reluctance to use opioids due to concerns about addiction or an overreliance on non-pharmacological treatments that may not be sufficient on their own.

5.2 Healthcare system limitations

5.2.1 Systemic barriers to effective pain management

- *Access to specialized care:* Many elderly patients have limited access to pain specialists, particularly in rural or underserved areas. This can lead to a reliance on primary care providers who may not have the expertise or resources to manage complex chronic pain cases effectively.

- *Time constraints and fragmented care:* The healthcare system often imposes time constraints on providers, making it difficult to conduct thorough pain assessments and develop comprehensive treatment plans. Additionally, care for elderly patients is often fragmented, with multiple providers managing different aspects of care. This can lead to inconsistencies in pain management strategies and a lack of coordinated care.

- *Insurance and cost barriers:* Financial constraints, including inadequate insurance coverage for pain management services (such as physical therapy, mental health services or alternative therapies), can limit the treatment options available to elderly patients. High out-of-pocket costs for medications or treatments can also deter patients from seeking or adhering to recommended pain management plans.

- *Long-term care facility challenges:* In nursing homes and other long-term care facilities, chronic pain is often under-recognized and undertreated due to staffing shortages, inadequate training of caregivers and the high prevalence of cognitive impairments among residents. These factors can contribute to insufficient pain management in these settings.

5.3 Patient and family education

5.3.1 The role of education in improving pain management

- *Empowering patients:* Education is key to empowering elderly patients to advocate for their pain management. By educating patients about the nature of chronic pain, available treatment options and the importance of reporting pain, healthcare providers can encourage more proactive pain management. This includes teaching patients about the potential benefits and risks of various treatments and helping them to make informed decisions.

- *Addressing myths and misconceptions:* Education can help dispel myths about pain and aging, such as the belief that pain is a normal part of getting older or that strong pain medications should be avoided at all costs. Providers should educate patients and their families about the difference between chronic and acute pain and the importance of managing chronic pain to prevent further physical and emotional deterioration.

- *Family involvement:* Involving family members in the education process is crucial, especially when the patient has cognitive impairments or other barriers to self-management. Families can play a vital role in monitoring pain, ensuring adherence to treatment plans and advocating for the patient's needs. Education should focus on teaching family members how to recognize signs of pain, how to communicate effectively with healthcare providers and how to support the patient in following their pain management plan.

- *Continuity of education:* Pain management education should be an ongoing process, integrated into every stage of care. This includes initial diagnosis, treatment planning and follow-up care. Educational materials should be tailored to the patient's cognitive level and include simple, clear instructions. Providing written materials, visual aids or even digital resources can reinforce key messages and improve understanding.

6. Policy and advocacy for pain management in the aging population the need for better policies

6.1 Addressing systemic barriers

- *Access to care:* There is a critical need for policies that ensure better access to pain management services for the elderly. This includes expanding coverage for non-pharmacological treatments such as physical therapy, mental health services and complementary therapies, which are often underutilized due to cost barriers. Policies should also focus on improving access to pain specialists, particularly in underserved areas.

- *Training and education for healthcare providers:* Effective pain management in the elderly requires specialized knowledge and skills. Policies should mandate better training for healthcare providers in geriatric pain management, including the use of comprehensive pain assessment tools, appropriate pharmacological management and the integration of non-pharmacological therapies. Continuing education programs and certification requirements could help bridge existing knowledge gaps.

- *Standardization of pain management protocols:* To reduce variability in care, there is a need for standardized protocols that are specifically tailored to the elderly. These protocols should be evidence-based and include guidelines for the assessment, treatment and monitoring of chronic pain in older adults. National guidelines could help ensure consistent, high-quality care across different healthcare settings.

6.2 Advocacy for patient rights and support

- *Raising awareness:* Advocacy efforts should focus on raising awareness about the prevalence and impact of chronic pain in the elderly. This includes educating the public, healthcare providers and policymakers about the unique challenges faced by older adults with chronic pain. Campaigns could highlight the importance of recognizing and treating pain as a serious health issue, rather than an inevitable consequence of aging.

- *Patient-centered care initiatives:* Policies should support the development of patient-centered care models that prioritize the needs and preferences of elderly patients. This includes promoting shared decision-making, where patients and their families are actively involved in the development of pain management plans. Advocacy efforts should push for policies that support the integration of care, ensuring that all aspects of a patient's pain and overall health are addressed.

- *Support for caregivers:* Recognizing the critical role that family caregivers play in managing chronic pain in the elderly, there is a need for policies that provide support and resources for caregivers. This could include education on pain management, respite care and financial support for those who care for elderly family members.

6.3 Legislative initiatives

- *Reforming prescription drug policies:* Given the risks associated with opioid use in the elderly, there is a need for balanced policies that both prevent misuse and ensure access to necessary pain relief. This includes advocating for reforms that promote the safe prescribing of opioids, as well as encouraging the development and use of alternative pain treatments. Legislative efforts could also focus on improving monitoring systems to prevent abuse while ensuring that elderly patients do not suffer from undertreated pain.

- *Funding for research and innovation:* Continued advocacy is needed to secure funding for research into chronic pain in the elderly. This includes support for clinical trials of new treatments, studies on the long-term effects of existing therapies and research into the most effective ways to integrate pharmacological and non-pharmacological treatments. Advocacy efforts should also push for increased funding for the development of technologies that can enhance pain management in this population.

DOI: http://dx.doi.org/10.5772/intechopen.1010202

7. Future directions

Ongoing research and innovation are crucial to advancing the management of chronic pain in the elderly, offering new hope for more effective and safer treatments. However, these advances must be supported by strong policies and advocacy efforts that address the systemic barriers to care and ensure that the unique needs of the aging population are met. By fostering an environment where both innovative treatments and comprehensive, patient-centered care are prioritized, we can improve the quality of life for elderly individuals living with chronic pain.

7.1 Ongoing research into new treatments and technologies pharmacological innovations

- *Targeted drug delivery systems:* Research is ongoing into more effective and safer drug delivery systems, such as transdermal patches, nanotechnology-based delivery systems and implantable pumps. These systems aim to provide consistent pain relief while minimizing systemic side effects, which is particularly important for the elderly who are often at higher risk of adverse drug reactions due to polypharmacy and comorbidities.

- *Novel analgesics:* The development of new classes of analgesics that target specific pain pathways with fewer side effects is a major focus. For example, research into selective ion channel blockers and monoclonal antibodies that target nerve growth factor (NGF) are showing promise for conditions like osteoarthritis and other forms of chronic pain. These therapies could offer pain relief with reduced risks compared to traditional NSAIDs or opioids.

- *Personalized medicine:* Advances in genomics and biomarkers are paving the way for personalized pain management. By identifying genetic variations that affect drug metabolism and pain perception, researchers hope to tailor treatments to the individual, optimizing efficacy and minimizing side effects. This approach is particularly valuable in the elderly, where inter-individual variability in drug response is often pronounced.

7.2 Non-pharmacological innovations

- *Neuromodulation technologies:* Technologies like spinal cord stimulation (SCS), transcranial magnetic stimulation (TMS) and deep brain stimulation (DBS) are being refined and studied for their effectiveness in treating chronic pain in the elderly. These technologies offer the potential for long-term pain relief by modulating pain pathways in the nervous system and ongoing research aims to enhance their efficacy, safety and accessibility for older adults.

- *Virtual reality (VR) and digital therapies:* VR-based pain management programs are being explored as non-invasive, drug-free options for chronic pain relief. These programs can offer immersive environments that distract from pain or provide cognitive-behavioral interventions more engagingly. Digital platforms that offer guided exercises, meditation and pain education are also being developed and tested specifically for the elderly population.

- *Regenerative medicine:* Research into regenerative therapies, such as stem cell therapy and platelet-rich plasma (PRP), is ongoing for conditions like osteoarthritis and degenerative disc disease. These therapies aim to repair or replace damaged tissues, potentially offering longer-term solutions to chronic pain. While still largely experimental, they hold promise for reducing reliance on traditional pain medications.

7.3 Integrative and complementary approaches

- *Mind-body interventions:* Research into the efficacy of mind-body interventions, such as mindfulness-based stress reduction (MBSR), tai chi and yoga, is expanding, with studies focusing on how these practices can be tailored for the elderly. These approaches are being integrated into broader pain management programs and are being evaluated for their ability to reduce pain, improve function and enhance quality of life without the risks associated with pharmacological treatments.

- *Nutritional and dietary interventions:* There is growing interest in how diet and specific nutritional supplements can influence pain and inflammation in the elderly. Research is exploring the role of anti-inflammatory diets, omega-3 fatty acids and other supplements in managing chronic pain, to offer safe and effective alternatives to traditional pain management strategies.

Acknowledgements

I acknowledge the use of ChatGPT-3.5 (Open AI, Available from: https://chat.openai.com/) to summarize challenges and barriers, policy and advocacy for pain management in the elderly.

Conflict of interest

P.B.A. declared no conflict of interest or disclosures.

DOI: http://dx.doi.org/10.5772/intechopen.1010202

Author details

Caroline Bozzetto Ambrosi[1] and Patricia Bozzetto Ambrosi[2,3]*

1 Clinical Medicine and Palliative Care, United Kingdom

2 European Academy of Neurology, France

3 Independent Clinical Neurology and Imaging Consultant, United Kingdom

*Address all correspondence to: patricia.ambrosi@icloud.com

References

[1] Dagnino APA, Campos MM. Chronic Pain in the Elderly: Mechanisms and Perspectives. Frontiers in Human Neuroscience. 3 Mar 2022;**16**:736688. DOI: 10.3389/fnhum.2022.736688

[2] Zis P, Daskalaki A, Bountouni I, Sykioti P, Varrassi G, Paladini A. Depression and chronic pain in the elderly: Links and management challenges. Clinical Interventions in Aging. 2017;**12**(12):709-720. Available from: https://www.ncbi.nlm.nih.gov/pmc/articles/PMC5407450/

[3] Wallace DC. The inevitability of growing old. Journal of Chronic Diseases. 1967;**20**(7):475-486

[4] Treede RD, Rief W, Barke A, Aziz Q, Bennett MI, Benoliel R, et al. Chronic pain as a symptom or a disease. Pain. 2019;**160**(1):19-27. Available from: https://journals.lww.com/pain/abstract/2019/01000/chronic_pain_as_a_symptom_or_a_disease the_iasp.3.aspx

[5] Molton IR, Terrill AL. Overview of persistent pain in older adults. The American Psychologist. 2014;**69**(2):197-207. Available from: https://www.apa.org/pubs/journals/releases/amp-a0035794.pdf

[6] Domenichiello AF, Ramsden CE. The silent epidemic of chronic pain in older adults. Progress in Neuro-Psychopharmacology and Biological Psychiatry. 2019;**93**(93):284-290

[7] Van der Meulen M, Rischer KM, González Roldán AM, Terrasa JL, Montoya P, Anton F. Age-related differences in functional connectivity associated with pain modulation. Neurobiology of Aging. 2024;**140**:1-11. Available from: https://www.sciencedirect.com/science/article/pii/S0197458024000794

[8] de Souza IMB, Sakaguchi TF, Yuan SLK, Matsutani LA, do Espírito-Santo AS, Pereira CAB, et al. Prevalence of low back pain in the elderly population: A systematic review. Clinics (Sao Paulo). Oct 28 2019;**74**:e789. DOI: 10.6061/clinics/2019/e789

[9] Saes-Silva E, Vieira YP, de Oliveira Saes M, Meucci RD, Aikawa P, Cousin E, et al. Epidemiology of chronic back pain among adults and elderly from Southern Brazil: A cross-sectional study. Brazilian Journal of Physical Therapy. 2021;**25**(3):344-351

[10] Cravello L, Di Santo S, Varrassi G, Benincasa D, Marchettini P, de Tommaso M, et al. Chronic pain in the elderly with cognitive decline: A narrative review. Pain and therapy. 2019;**8**(1):53-65. Available from: https://link.springer.com/article/10.1007%2Fs40122-019-0111-7#citeas

[11] Stokes AC, Xie W, Lundberg DJ, Hempstead K, Zajacova A, Zimmer Z, et al. Increases in BMI and chronic pain for US adults in midlife, 1992 to 2016. SSM - Population Health. 2020;**12**:100644

[12] Kirubakaran S, Dongre A. Chronic musculoskeletal pain among elderly in rural Tamil Nadu: Mixed-method study. Journal of Family Medicine and Primary Care. 2019;**8**(1):77

[13] Mallon T, Eisele M, König HH, Brettschneider C, Roehr S, Pabst A, et al. Lifestyle aspects as a predictor of pain among oldest-old primary care patients—A longitudinal cohort study. Clinical Interventions in Aging. 2019;**14**:1881-1888

[14] De Lucia A, Perlini C, Chiarotto A, Pachera S, Pasini I, Del Piccolo L,

et al. eHealth-integrated psychosocial and physical interventions for chronic pain in older adults: Scoping review. Journal of Medical Internet Research. 2024;**26**:e55366. Available from: https://www.jmir.org/2024/1/e55366/

[15] Tinnirello A, Mazzoleni S, Santi C. Chronic pain in the elderly: Mechanisms and distinctive features. Biomolecules. 2021;**11**(8):1256

[16] Guo J, Huang X, Dou L, Yan M, Shen T, Tang W, et al. Aging and aging-related diseases: From molecular mechanisms to interventions and treatments. Signal Transduction and Targeted Therapy. 2022;**7**(1):391. Available from: https://www.nature.com/articles/s41392-022-01251-0

[17] Yezierski RP. The effects of age on pain sensitivity: Preclinical studies. Pain Medicine. 2012;**13 Suppl 2**(Suppl. 2):S27-S36. DOI: 10.1111/j.1526-4637.2011.01311.x

[18] Cohen SP, Mao J. Neuropathic pain: Mechanisms and their clinical implications. BMJ. 2014;**348**:f7656. DOI: 10.1136/bmj.f7656

[19] Fang XX, Zhai MN, Zhu M, He C, Wang H, Wang J, et al. Inflammation in pathogenesis of chronic pain: Foe and friend. Molecular Pain. 2023;**19**:174480692311781

[20] Ji RR, Chamessian A, Zhang YQ. Pain regulation by non-neuronal cells and inflammation. Science. 2016;**354**(6312):572-577. Available from: https://science.sciencemag.org/content/354/6312/572.full

[21] Ali A, Arif AW, Bhan C, Kumar D, Malik MB, Sayyed Z, et al. Managing chronic pain in the elderly: An overview of the recent therapeutic advancements. Cureus. 2018;**10**(9):e3293. Available from: https://www.ncbi.nlm.nih.gov/pmc/articles/PMC6235641/

[22] Guidelines For Pain Management In The Elderly. 1st ed. 2018. Available from: https://www.moh.gov.my/moh/resources/Penerbitan/Program%20Bebas%20Kesakitan/Garis%20Panduan/Geriatric_Pain_Management_2018_(1st_Ed.)_.pdf

[23] National Institute for Health and Care Excellence. Find Guidance | NICE. NICE; 2024

[24] Royal College of Physicians. British Geriatrics Society and British Pain Society the Assessment of Pain in Older People: National Guidelines, Concise Guidance to Good Practice Series, No 8. London: RCP; 2007. Available from: http://britishpainsociety.org/book_pain_older_people.pdf

[25] Abdulla A, Adams N, Bone M, et al. Guidance on the management of pain in older people. Age and Ageing. 2013;**42**(Suppl. 1):1-57. Available from: http://ageing.oxfordjournals.org/content/42/suppl_1.toc

[26] McDonald D, Shea M, Rose L, et al. The effect of pain question phrasing on older adult pain information. Journal of Pain and Symptom Management. 2009;**37**:1050-1060

[27] Merskey H, Bogduk N, editors. Classification of Chronic Pain: Descriptions of Chronic Pain Syndromes and Definition of Pain Terms. International Association for the Study of Pain; 1994. Available from: http://www.iasp-pain.org/les/Content/ContentFolders/Publications2/FreeBooks/Classication-of-Chronic-Pain.pdf

[28] Bindu S, Mazumder S, Bandyopadhyay U. Non-steroidal

anti-inflammatory drugs (NSAIDs) and organ damage: A current perspective. Biochemical Pharmacology. 2020;**180**(1):114147

[29] National Institutes of Health. Pathways to Prevention Workshop: The Role of Opioids in the Treatment of Chronic Pain. Executive Summary [Internet]. 2014. Available from: https://prevention.nih.gov/sites/default/files/documents/programs/p2p/ODPPainPanelStatementFinal_10-02-14.pdf

[30] Knotkova H, Hamani C, Sivanesan E, Beuffe MFEL, Moon JY, Cohen SP, et al. Neuromodulation for chronic pain. The Lancet. 2021;**397**(10289):2111-2124

[31] Ambrose KR, Golightly YM. Physical exercise as non-pharmacological treatment of chronic pain: Why and when. Best Practice & Research. Clinical Rheumatology. 2015;**29**(1):120-130. Available from: https://www.ncbi.nlm.nih.gov/pmc/articles/PMC4534717/

[32] Bishop MD, Torres-Cueco R, Gay CW, Lluch-Girbés E, Beneciuk JM, Bialosky JE. What effect can manual therapy have on a patient's pain experience? Pain Management. 2015;**5**(6):455-464. Available from: https://www.ncbi.nlm.nih.gov/pmc/articles/PMC4976880/

[33] Lim JA, Choi SH, Lee WJ, Jang JH, Moon JY, Kim YC, et al. Cognitivebehavioral therapy for patients with chronic pain: Implications of gender differences in empathy. Medicine (Baltimore). Jun 2018;**97**(23):e10867. DOI: 10.1097/MD.0000000000010867. PMID: 29879022; PMCID: PMC5999451

[34] Wielgosz J, Kral TRA, Perlman DM, Mumford JA, Wager TD, Lutz A, et al. Neural Signatures of Pain Modulation in Short-Term and Long-Term Mindfulness Training: A Randomized Active-Control Trial. The American Journal of Psychiatry. Oct 2022;**179**(10):758-767. DOI: 10.1176/appi.ajp.21020145. Epub 2022 Jul 28. Erratum in: Am J Psychiatry. Oct 2022;179(10):767. DOI: 10.1176/appi.ajp.21020145correction

[35] Vickers AJ, Vertosick EA, Lewith G, MacPherson H, Foster NE, Sherman KJ, et al. Acupuncture for chronic pain: Update of an individual patient data meta-analysis. The Journal of Pain. 2018;**19**(5):455-474. Available from: https://www.jpain.org/article/S1526-5900(17)30780-0/fulltext

[36] Mann DJ, Mattox R. Chiropractic management of a patient with chronic pain in a federally qualified health center: A case report. Journal of Chiropractic Medicine. 2018;**17**(2):117-120

[37] Buesing S, Costa M, Schilling JM, Moeller-Bertram T. Vitamin B12 as a treatment for pain. Pain Physician. 2019;**22**(1):E45-E52. Available from: https://pubmed.ncbi.nlm.nih.gov/30700078/

[38] Gatchel RJ, McGeary DD, McGeary CA, Lippe B. Interdisciplinary chronic pain management: past, present, and future. American Psychologist. Feb-Mar 2014;**69**(2):119-130. DOI: 10.1037/a0035514

Chapter 7

The Role of Exercise Therapy in the Management of Parkinson's Disease

Terry Jeremy Ellapen, Brink M. Ntjana, Chenelle Ribeiro-Wagener and Yvonne Paul

Abstract

Parkinson's disease (PD) is a progressive neurological pathology characterized by the loss of dopaminergic neurons in the midbrain. The disease can be either genetic or non-genetic in etiology. Parkinson's disease is characterized by bradykinesia, muscular rigidity, resting tremors, and postural instability. Although empirical scientific evidence hints that regular exercise therapy diminishes the symptoms of PD, greater awareness of this therapeutic modality is needed to better manage the pathology. This chapter will describe the beneficial role of exercise therapy in the management of PD through recent clinical empirical evidence. Further the chapter will describe the general exercise plan for PD patient rehabilitation and an example of contemporary exercises prescribed to PD patients. Finally, a brief description of prospective research endeavors needed to understand the effects of exercise therapy in reversing the PD pathophysiology.

Keywords: Parkinson disease, elderly, exercise therapy, strengthening, flexibility, aerobic exercise, cardiometabolic diseases

1. Introduction

Human gerontology is the study of the aging process, which extends from maturation (adulthood) toward old age (late adulthood). Geriatrics is a branch of clinical medicine concerned with the diagnosis, treatment, and rehabilitation of older people. Human life undergoes the following stages of development: (i) infancy, (ii) early childhood, (iii) middle childhood, (iv) adolescence, (v) early adulthood, (vi) middle adulthood, and (vii) late adulthood. Human physiology and anatomy changes over the course of one's life, characterize different stages in the individual's life. From birth to 21 years, the person muscular, skeletal, nervous, cognitive, cardiovascular, and respiratory systems are developing in size strength, endurance, and prowess. Chronologically from 20 to 40 years, the individual is in their peak physiological and anatomical functional state, and thereafter their physiological and anatomical abilities start to decline. A person's cognitive prowess is at prime function during the age of 40–60 years and thereafter starts to decline.

During the last century, medical and rehabilitative medicine has made numerous advances in the field geriatric health care, which has inevitably lengthened the average human beings' mortality. In 2000, the average human life expectancy was 66.8 years, which has increased to 73.4 years in 2019. Although the nomenclature geriatric is attached to the age of 65 years and beyond, colloquially individuals aged 60 years are considered as elderly or senior citizens. The World Health Organization in 2022 reported that the international geriatric populace (60 years and older) is anticipated to expand from 900 million as measured in 2015 to two billion by 2050 [1]. The age strata of 80 years and older is anticipated to expand their number from 125 million in 2015 to 434 million by 2050 [1].

Aging is synonymous with a declining in cognitive and physiological functioning [2]. Fundamental geriatric changes affect human physiology and anatomy are characterized by reduced cardiorespiratory endurance, muscular strength and endurance, coordination, and poor proprioception [2]. These adverse manifestations associated with the aging process lead to an inferior quality of life and a greater predisposing risk of falling and diseases [3]. The elderly are also predisposed to variety of neurological diseases such strokes (cerebrovascular incidents), Alzheimer's disease, Parkinson's disease (PD), multiple sclerosis, and cerebral palsy. Alzheimer's disease is a type of dementia. The initial symptoms of this disease are mild memory loss leading to inability to carry out a conversation and inappropriate behavior. Alzheimer's disease affects anatomical structures of the brain that control memory, thought, and language processing [4]. Multiple sclerosis is a pathology whereby the person's own immune system attacks the myelin sheath, which covers the brain and optic nerve cells and spinal cord. The damage to myelin sheaths causes memory loss, muscle weakness, numbness, and blindness [5]. Cerebral palsy is a result of damage to the brain, impacting the individual's posture and movement. Often these pathologies are clustered together because of their neurological deficits to human physiological functioning [6]. This chapter exclusively focuses on Parkinson's disease (PD) and the adjunct value of exercise therapy in its treatment plan.

This chapter will describe the beneficial role of exercise is to PD patients. A synopsis of the pathophysiology of PD, signs and symptoms of the disease, and justification for the inclusion of exercise therapy in the treatment of PD is presented. The various components of a physical examination commonly used among clinical exercise physiologists, physiotherapists, and biokineticists are described. Using the information gathered from the physical examination exercise, therapists will prescribe structured physical activity and exercise programme. Finally, direction for prospective empirical research in the field of exercise therapy as a treatment intervention for PD patients will be described.

2. Parkinson's disease

Parkinson's disease (PD) is an advancing neurodegenerative pathology distinguishable by resting tremor, muscle rigidity, bradykinesia, postural instability, loss of proprioception, and gait abnormalities. This pathology was initially described by Dr. James Parkinson in 1817. Parkinson's disease is the second most prevalent neurological disease after Alzheimer's disease [7]. Nussbuam and colleagues reported that the disease has a prevalence of approximately one percent among individuals aged 65–69 years and steadily rises to three percent among individuals aged 80 years of age and older. It is expected that the incidence of PD will upsurge 30% of most geriatric populations by 2030 [8]. This increase in PD patient number will result in direct and indirect financial implications for the patient, their family, and society [9].

DOI: http://dx.doi.org/10.5772/intechopen.1006114

2.1 Signs and symptoms of Parkinson's disease

A symptom is a sensation of disease apparent to the patient themselves. A symptom is commonly described as the pathological sensation the patient experience, which is not felt by others. A sign is the display of disease that the physician can identify. Parkinson's disease has been identified as a progressive disease that attacks the nervous system and the parts of the body controlled by the nervous system. Ridgel and Pollock identified resting tremors, bradykinesia, and muscle rigidity as cardinal signs of Parkinson's disease [10]. A brief description of each sign will be provided in order of most prevalent among PD patients.

- Parkinson's disease tremor is the first motor sign of the disorder, which is most evident when the individual is at rest, and therefore, is commonly referred to as resting tremor. These tremors diminish in intensity while the person is asleep and are difficult to distinguish when the person is active. It is common occurrence to observe the person's hand, shaking or trembling while sitting [10]. This sign starts slowly and progressively intensifies. Tremors generally start in the person's hands and are often described as "pill-rolling". However, tremors are not limited to the hands and spread to other parts of the body, including the jaw, lower lip, and leg. These tremors may disturb daily activities such as bathing, dressing, shaving, writing, and many other tasks that require fine motor coordination [10].

- Bradykinesia is a clinical term referring to slowness of movement. It is one of the prime signs of PD. Epidemiologists have attributed that sarcopenia, tremors, and muscle rigidity in part contribute to this symptom of PD. The initial signs of bradykinesia include reduced involuntary movements such as eye blinking or normal arm swinging when you walk. Progressive signs include difficulty to initiate the sit-to-stand maneuver out of a chair and loss of facial expressions. Bradykinesia is synonymous with the following biomechanical terminology: akinesia (the inability to move your muscles voluntarily) and hypokinesia (slow and small movements, such as a shuffling gait) [11].

- Muscle rigidity refers to muscle stiffness or contractures. Muscle contractures are generally caused by lack of muscle extensibility due to physical inactivity and flexibility exercises. Muscle rigidity is associated with muscle pain, spasms cramps, and poor proprioception. Common anatomical joints of rigidity include cervical vertebrae (neck), radiocarpal (wrist), ulnohumeral (elbow), tibiofemoral (knee), and talocrural (ankle) [12].

- The postural changes include cervical postural syndrome, protracted scapula and shoulders, kyphosis, and loss of normal lumbar lordotic vertebral curve. Clinical exercise physiologists, physiotherapists, and biokineticists attribute postural instability to muscle contractures and asymmetry. Postural instability contributes to the patient's inability to maintain their balance and proprioception. The addition of postural instability increases the risk of falls [13].

- Loss of proper gait kinematics is often observed among PD patients, manifested by reduced stride length and foot clearance, and loss of heel to toe foot landing kinematics. These biomechanical gait abnormalities allow the PD patient to display a shuffling gait. Many PD patients have a flexed posture, which moves them quicker out of their base of support, resulting in the person taking quicker but shorter steps with inability to stop and balance. This increases the risk of falls. The forward propulsion caused by the deviant posture and the quick steps is often referred to as festination. Many PD patients natural arm swing during walking is lost or slowed [14].

- Poor proprioception is common among PD patients caused by the decreased postural reflexes. If patients are perturbed beyond the base of support, the person is unable to regain their balance in their base of support and will fall. The incidence of falls is high among PD patients [10, 14].

2.2 Rationale for the inclusion of regular physical activity and exercise as a major component of daily living among the elderly

The benefits of habitual physical activity, sport, and exercise are widespread, which included increased sport performance, enhanced physiological functioning, decreased risk, and onset of chronic diseases such as cardiovascular and metabolic, cancer, depression, arthritis, and osteoporosis, and this leads to increased longevity [11]. Physical activity also improve cognitive physiology by altering neuroplasticity and neurochemistry. The primary goals of habitual physical activity and exercise for the geriatric populace were aimed to improve their cardiorespiratory conditioning and longevity. The American College of Sports Medicine position stand statement in 2009 advocated that the elderly can also enjoy the exercise induce benefits to arrest the hypokinetic diseases associated with advanced aging [12]. A balanced exercise programme for the elderly must include aerobic (cardiovascular) activity, flexibility, proprioception, and muscle strength and endurance (**Table 1**). The integration of habitual physical activity and exercise into the lifestyle of the geriatric population are premised on the following:

- Empirical research has identified that osteoporosis, arthritis, fractures, mobility impairment, and poor functionality are associated with reduced muscle extensibility and joint range of motion, which can be addressed by flexibility and muscle strengthening exercises [13, 14]. Sarcopenia and osteoporosis which are prevalent among the elderly can be rehabilitated through resistance muscle strengthening and endurance exercises [13, 14].

- Aging associated physiological decline has been likened to disuse and physical inactivity, which has swayed clinical exercise physiologists to believe that the manner in which we age is determined by our physical activity regularity and intensity.

- The onset of chronic diseases has been associated with advancing of age. The adherence to exercise therapy has demonstrated to be a powerful treatment modality to arrest the progress of various chronic diseases such as cardiovascular diseases, metabolic diseases, sarcopenia, and osteoporosis [15, 16].

- Orthodox medical management of hypokinetic diseases plaguing the aged does not address a physical inactive lifestyle which is responsible for much of the disability and morbidity of the disease [17].

DOI: http://dx.doi.org/10.5772/intechopen.1006114

Training method	Frequency	Intensity	Duration	Mode	Progression	Important consideration
Cardiorespiratory	3 days/wk	60–80% VO_2 R or HRR or RPE: 11–13	30 min continuous or accumulated	Leg ergometry, walking/jogging, swimming	Slow, programme personalized	Improve walking economy, gait and balance
Resistance	2–3 days/wk	40–50% of 1RM for novice, 60–70% 1RM for advance	1 set or more of 8–12 reps for novice	Machine and free weights, resistance bands	Start 1 set: 8–15 reps of 1RM, progress to 2 sets of 8–12 reps	↑ muscle strength and endurance. ↓ muscle fatigue. ↑ ADL
Range of Motion	1–7 days/wk	Stretch to point of mild discomfort	10–30 sec	Slow static stretches all major muscle groups	Starts with static stretch moving to functional	↑ proprioception, ROM.

VO_2R: VO_2 Reserve, HRR: Heart Rate Reserve, 1RM: one repetition maximum, wk.: week, ROM; range of motion.

Table 1.
Exercise therapy plan for Parkinson's disease patients [10].

- Many pathophysiological abnormalities associated with hypokinetic diseases and aging can be addressed with regular structure clinical evidence-based exercise therapy.

- Regular physical activity is considered a protective mechanism to combat the pathogenesis of noncommunicable diseases (cerebrovascular events, cardiovascular disease, diabetes mellitus, and cancer). Regular physical activity and exercise has also been associated with enhanced mental health and quality of life and wellbeing. Mental health includes cognitive function and psychological and social well-being [18].

2.3 Scientific justification of exercise therapy in the management of Parkinson's disease

Habitual adherence to exercise therapy and physical activity among PD patients has demonstrated deceleration the pathological progress, reduced the discomfort and pain, prolonged independence to mobility activities (such as balance and gait) and improved sleeping behavior, attitude to life, and overall enhanced quality of life. This subsection will describe the effects of regular exercise and physical activity had on PD patient in terms on the cognitive skills, balance, gait, and pain.

- Murray et al. described the beneficial impact of exercise on cognition through neuroprotection and neurogenesis [11, 19]. Murray and colleagues illustrated that different modes of exercise, such as aerobic, dance, and resistance, were able to improve cognitive function [11, 19]. The limitations of their findings were the dose response of exercise: amount (volume), intensity, and duration of exercise [11, 19]. Ahlskog concurred that physical activity enhances cognition and diminished the risk of dementia and mild cognitive impairment [20]. He further advocates that regular exercise and physical activity during human beings' midlife reduces their risk of developing PD [20]. Habitual vigorous exercise and physical activity decrease medical refractory motor problems associated with PD. Ahlskog reported that exercise and physical activity increased brain-derived neurotrophic factor, which protected the brain from the dopaminergic neurotoxins [20].

- Kolk and King reported that the balance and gait challenges among PD patients are difficult to manage by the pharmacological treatment alone. They reported that exercise and physical activity has the probability to improve motor deficits of PD [21]. The motor deficits include muscle strength, balance, and gait. Cholewa et al. and Kluding et al. reinforced Kolk and King postulations [21–23]. Cholewa and colleagues reported that bi-weekly exercise rehabilitation persisting for a minimum of an hour was able to improve joint range of motion and muscle extensibility (combating muscle rigidity/contractures), thereby improving balance and gait. Kluding et al. concurred Cholewa et al. findings [22, 23].

- Allen and colleagues reported that 85% of PD patients experience pain daily, which contributes to insomnia, depression, and reduced quality of life [24]. The symptom of pain is normally managed through the pharmacological prescription of analgesics combined with dopaminergic agents. Allen and colleagues proposed that regular exercise and physical activity can diminish pain by influencing the neuroplasticity (anatomical and physiological re-organization of the brain in response to environmental changes) and neuro-restoration (regeneration of damaged neurons) by increasing brain neurotrophic factors, angiogenesis, synaptic strength, and the body's immune response [24]. It was postulated that these altered responses were beneficial to change the central processing of pain. Allen and colleagues postulated that exercise activated the dopaminergic neurons, which initiated an anti-nociceptive role, suppressing nociceptive signaling and thereby reduced the severity of pain [24]. Fayyaz and colleagues postulate that regular exercise and physical activity can reduce pain among PD patients by activating the non-dopaminergic pain inhibitor pathways [25].

- The effects of cardiopulmonary rehabilitation on the aerobic capacity, cardiovascular and pulmonary health are limited. It is advised that the clinicians should be cautious when rehabilitating PD patients. Cardiopulmonary exercise intensity evidence of the effects of aerobic exercise on PD patients is slow due the rapid fatigue displayed by patients. However, moderate intensity cardiopulmonary exercises are tolerated and improve quality of life [10, 11]. However, the incidence of cardiometabolic comorbidities among PD patients has been reported [26, 27]. Many PD patients have been identified has being obese, diabetic, and hypertensive [27]. The common pathophysiology of these cardiometabolic pathologies has been identified due to oxidative stress and chronic inflammation [28]. Regular physical activity (lightest intensity) at the leisure time has been associated with diminished risk of cardiovascular diseases and cerebrovascular incidents [28]. Empirical literature has demonstrated that leisure-time physical activity has an inverse relationship with the progression of PD and cardiometabolic comorbidities [29]. Shih and colleagues recommend moderate to vigorous intensity activities lower the cardiometabolic risk and disease progression of PD [29]. Potashkin and colleagues identified that individuals who have persistently exercised from their early life lower the risk of PD and reduce the severity of the disease [30]. Mak and colleagues suggest that the physiological mechanism by which regular physical activity reduces PD risk is due to increased neuroplasticity and brain-derived neurotrophic factors [11, 31]. Real et al. also reported that the lowered risk of PD attributed to exercise is due to reduction chronic neuroinflammation [32].

2.4 Physical examination

Exercise clinical physiologists, physiotherapists, and biokineticists should complete a thorough history and comprehensive neurological and orthopedic evaluation. During their neurological physical examinations, clinicians should review PD patients resting tremors, bradykinesia, muscle rigidity, postural deviations, and biomechanics of motion (gait). These symptoms will be described.

- To identify the presence of resting tremors, request the PD patient to sit placing the hands onto the lap. Stanley and Protas recommended that the PD patient recite a few sentences or count in multiples of 2 s, 5 s, 7 s [33]. The patient's focus on the mental task allows the presence of the resting tremors to become more evident. An alternate test would observe the person drink out of cup. If the act of picking the cup, moving the cup their mouth, drinking the fluid, and returning the cup is coupled with shaking, this would be positive for presence of tremors [33].

- To evaluate the presence of bradykinesia, request the patient to sit having both hands placed on their lap. Then ask the patient to supinate and pronate the forearm are quickly as possible for a 30 second duration. If the PD patient has bradykinesia, the quality of the required motor task will deteriorate within a few seconds. Other possible signs may include reduced range of motion, slowing of movement. Complete both hands [33].

- To establish the presence of muscle rigidity, the clinician should grasp the patient's wrist and shake them, up and down. If ease of movement is noticed, rigidity is absence. Thereafter patient should be requested to flex and extend the ulnohumeral (elbow), acetabulofemoral (hip), tibiofemoral (knee), and talocrural (ankle) joints, observing for ease of movement. The vertebrae (cervical, thoracic, and lumbar) must be observed for ease of movement in the frontal, sagittal, and transverse planes to rule out muscle rigidity [33]. Goniometry to measure joints of the ulnohumeral, acetabulofemoral, tibiofemoral, and talocrural joints is also advised. Clinician must identify specific loss of joint range of motion to prescribe rehabilitative programme.

- Parkinson's disease patients should undergo a postural screening. The clinician should be vigilant for cervical postural syndrome, thoracic hyperkyphosis, reduced lordosis, excessive anterior pelvic tilt, and flexed tibiofemoral joint in the sagittal plane. In the frontal plane, clinician should observe for scoliosis and protracted scapulae [33]. Cervical postural syndrome is characterized by a protruding chin and protracted/rounded scapula [34]. Thoracic hyperkyphosis is a clinical term referring to the excessive curvature of the thoracic vertebrae which appears as a rounded upper back [35]. Reduced lumbar lordosis is the loss of lumbar vertebrae natural inward curvature to become straighter, and thereby the lumbar vertebrae appears flatter. Anterior pelvic tilt is a postural condition where the person's pelvis is rotated or tilted anteriorly/forward. Scoliosis is a sideways curvature of the vertebrae. Flexed tibiofemoral is the appearance of a slight bend at the knee joint.

- Gait analyses involve reviewing the quality (coordination of movement) of the hip, knee, ankle, and foot during the stance and swing phases. Further the clinician should be vigilant for slow or absence arm swing during gait analyses.

2.5 Exercise and physical activity prescription

Clinical exercise physiologists, physiotherapists, and biokineticists base their structured physical activity and exercise prescription on the Hoehen and Yahr Classification. Parkinson's disease patients who fall into the Hoehn and Yahr Class 1 and 2 can comply with American College of Sports Medicine (ACSM) Guidelines [5]. However, PD patients categorized as Classes 3 and higher should comply with the

Basic CDD4 Recommendations for Parkinson's Diseased Patient modification. The fundamental goal of exercise therapy for PD patients is to improve one's quality of life. Their exercise programme should include the following components:

i. Flexibility

ii. Aerobic conditioning

iii. Strengthening

iv. Neuromuscular coordination-skill

v. Functional training.

The flexibility exercise prescription should be followed on a daily basis, starting with slow static stretching (**Table 1**). Each stretch should be maintained for a minimum of 20 seconds to comply with neurophysiological reflex guide. Slow static stretches maintained for 10 seconds and longer increases muscle length and eliminates the risk of injury. Resistance (or strength) training should be completed between two and three exercise sessions per week (**Table 1**). Resistance of the strength training varies for from 40 to 50% for novices, while more aggressive intensity of 60–70% for seasoned exercisers. Patients should complete one set of eight repetitions for each major muscle group when initially beginning a clinical exercise regime. Thereafter, as strength and muscle endurance increases, patients can increase to two sets of more repetitions (not exceeding 15) (**Table 1**). Resistance training should involve the use of elastic bands, machines, and/or free weights (dumbbells and barbells). Cardiorespiratory training aims to improve endurance, which improve walking kinematics and economy of motion (**Table 1**). Equipment that can be used includes leg ergometry, walking, jogging, and swimming. Cardiorespiratory exercise duration should last a maximum of 30 minutes. Initially patients can start with accumulated durations within a day to equate to 30 minutes if they cannot complete 30 minutes continuously (**Table 1**). Cardiorespiratory exercises should be completed a minimum of 3 days per week (**Table 1**).

Table 1 describes the general exercise therapy plan for PD patients, while **Table 2** provides examples of exercises that PD patients can perform.

2.6 Direction of prospective research

Parkinson's disease and cardiometabolic diseases share common pathophysiological mechanism such as chronic inflammation, lipid metabolism, oxidative stress, and insulin resistance in its disease progress [5, 10, 11]. Regular structured clinical exercise therapy has illustrated that the shared cardiometabolic modifiable risk factors among PD patients can be effectively managed [5, 10, 11]. However, the adequate dose response to bring about these therapeutic changes needs further investigation. The reliability of the positive effects of prolonged exercises such as aerobic, strengthening, flexibility, and proprioception reducing the signs and symptoms and disease progression is needed. Further empirical investigation of how regular structure exercise therapy as part of a multidisciplinary medical managing PD is needed.

Aerobic exercises (5–30 minutes)			
Walking with rail support (low intensity: 40% of heart rate reserve)	**Leg cycling (low intensity) (40% of heart rate reserve)**	**Arm ergometry (low intensity) (30% of heart rate reserve)**	
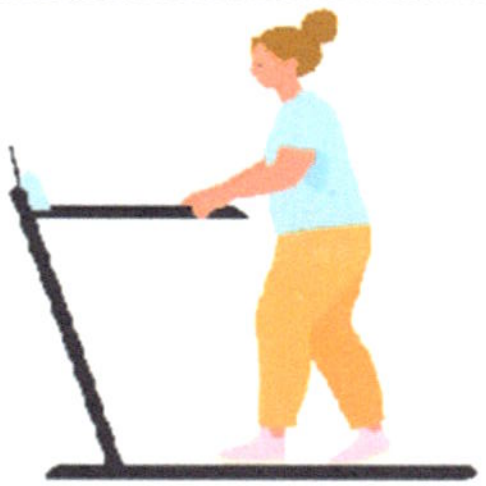	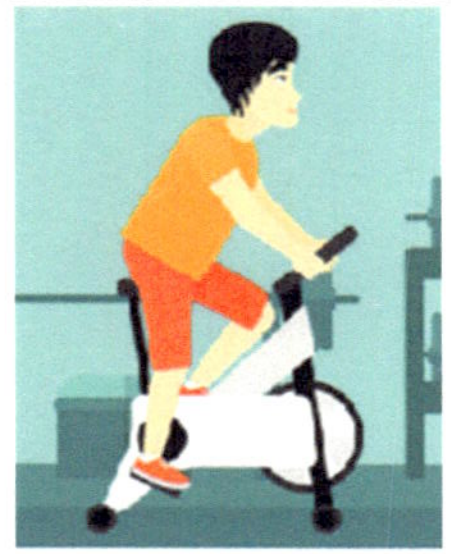	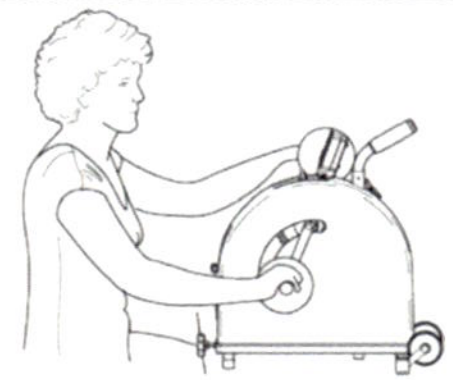	
Flexibility exercises (4 reps: static stretches – hold for 20 seconds)			
Neck flexion/extension	**Biceps/triceps stretch**	**Shoulder**	**Chest**
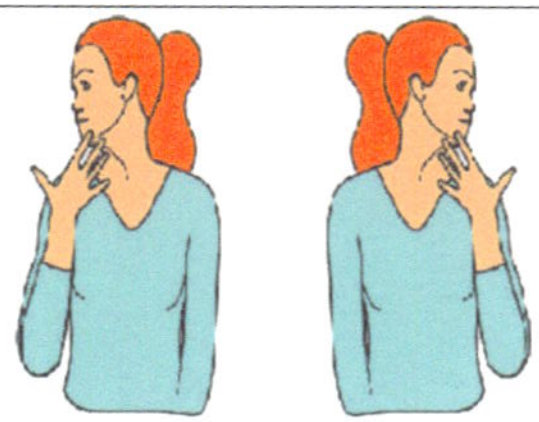	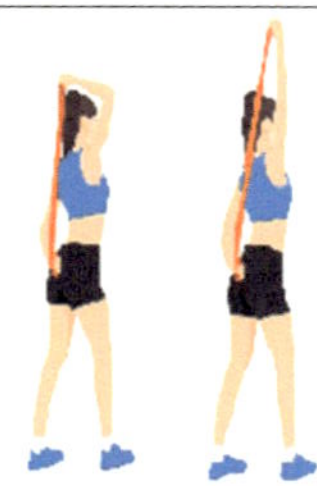	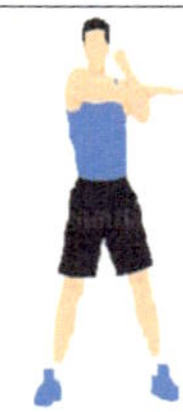	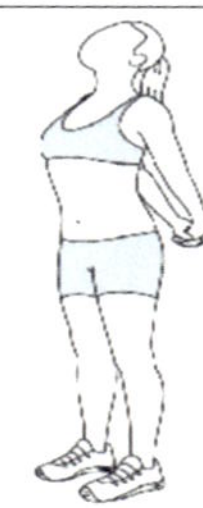

DOI: http://dx.doi.org/10.5772/intechopen.1006114

Aerobic exercises (5–30 minutes)			
Walking with rail support (low intensity: 40% of heart rate reserve)	**Leg cycling (low intensity) (40% of heart rate reserve)**	**Arm ergometry (low intensity) (30% of heart rate reserve)**	
Cat back	**Hip flexor/quadriceps**	**Hamstrings**	**Gastrocnemius**
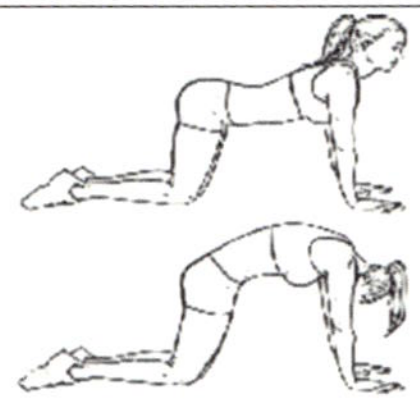	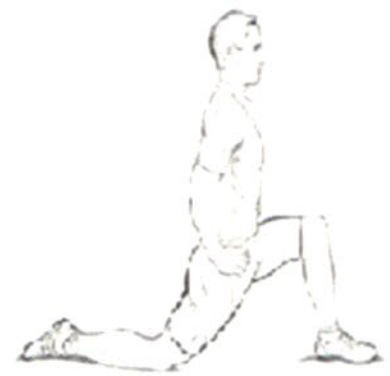	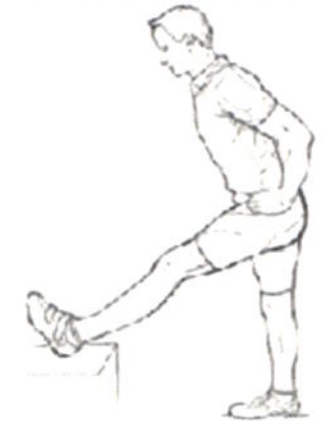	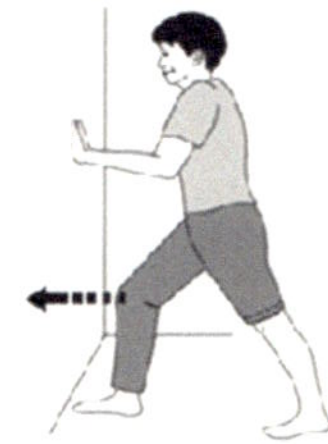
Soleus	**Lower back**	**Lateral obliques**	**Hip rotators**
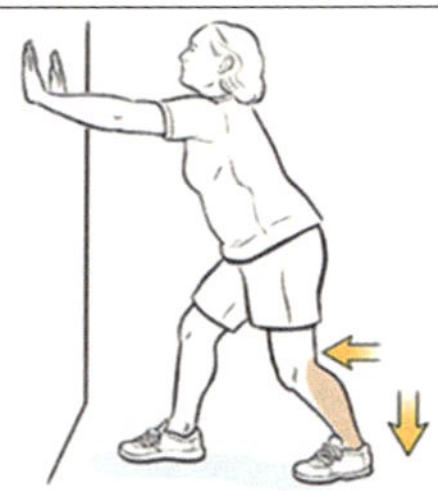	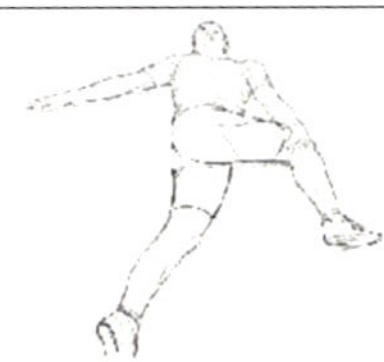	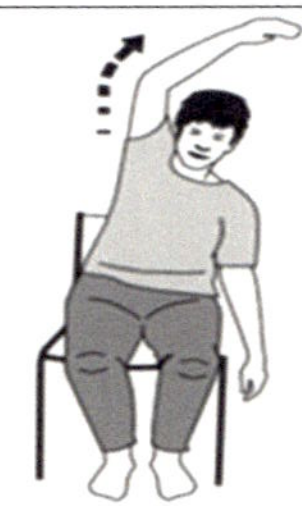	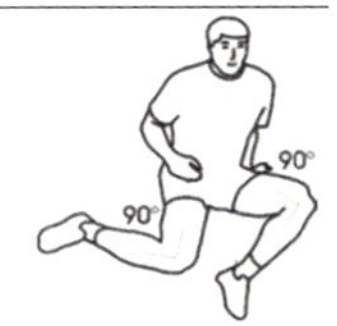
Strengthening exercises (2 sets × 10 reps)			

Aerobic exercises (5–30 minutes)		
Walking with rail support (low intensity: 40% of heart rate reserve)	Leg cycling (low intensity) (40% of heart rate reserve)	Arm ergometry (low intensity) (30% of heart rate reserve)
Shoulder shrug	Shoulder press	Lateral raises / Bent over flyes
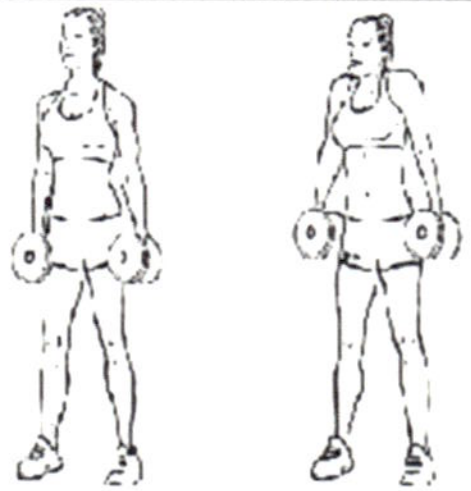	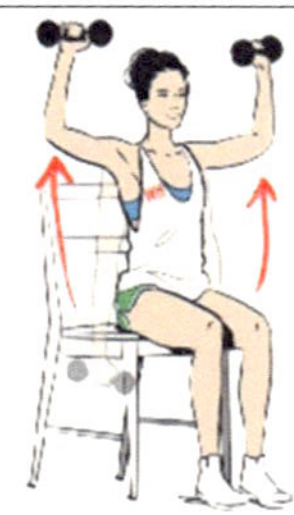	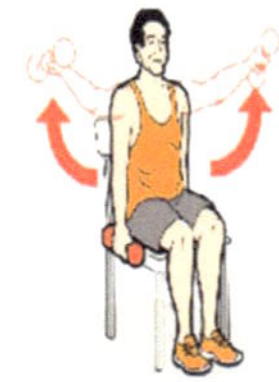 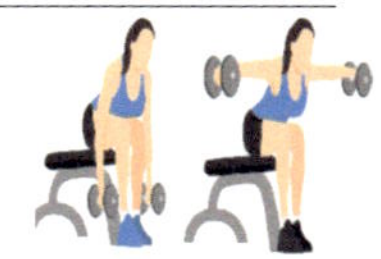
Seated trunk rotations	Calf raises	Straight leg raises
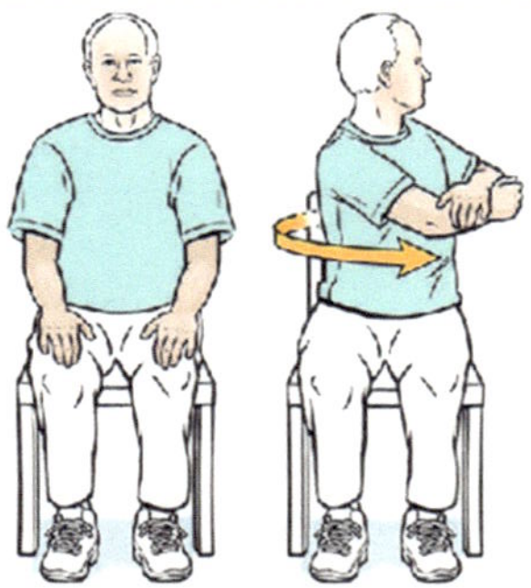	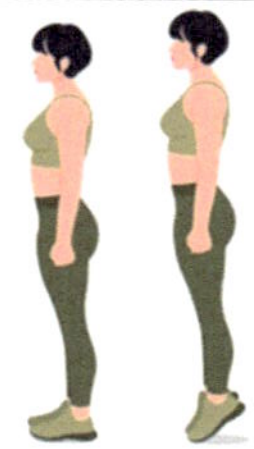	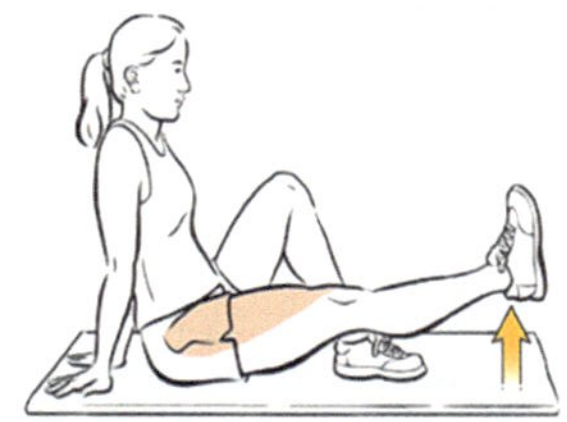
Wall push-ups	Wall angles	Wall squats

DOI: http://dx.doi.org/10.5772/intechopen.1006114

Aerobic exercises (5–30 minutes)		
Walking with rail support (low intensity: 40% of heart rate reserve)	**Leg cycling (low intensity) (40% of heart rate reserve)**	**Arm ergometry (low intensity) (30% of heart rate reserve)**
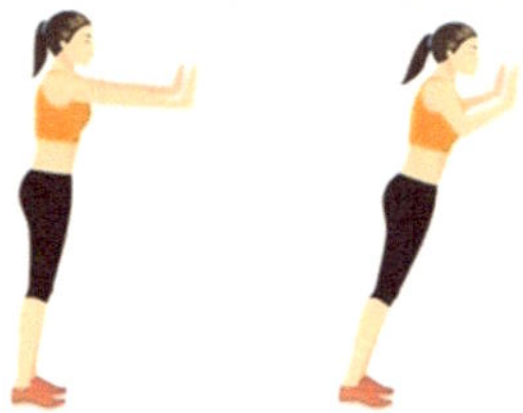	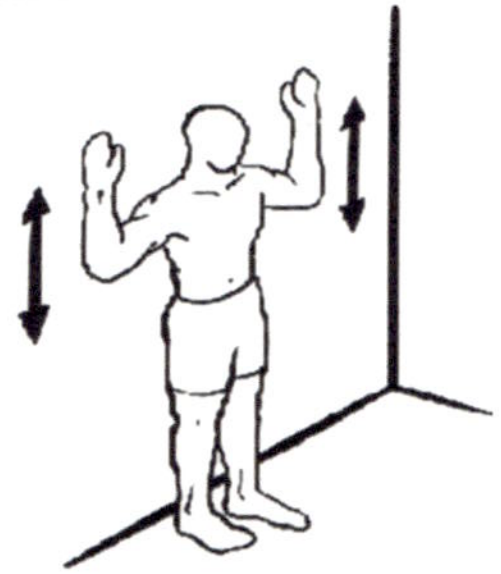	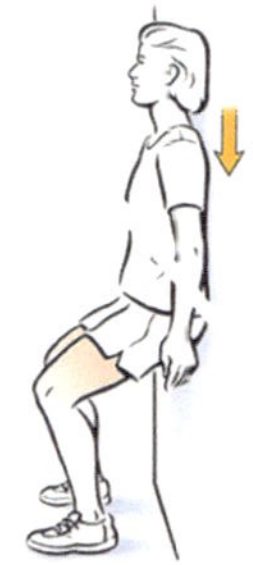
Balance and proprioception exercises (2 repetitions)		
Tandem walking	**Backward walking**	**Stalk stand**
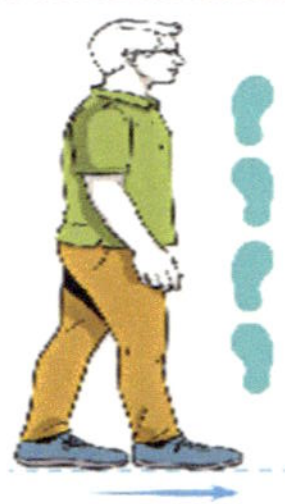	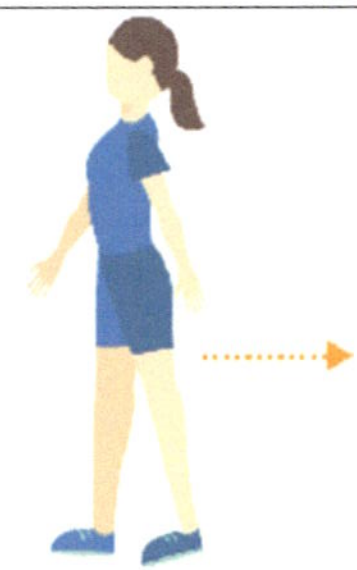	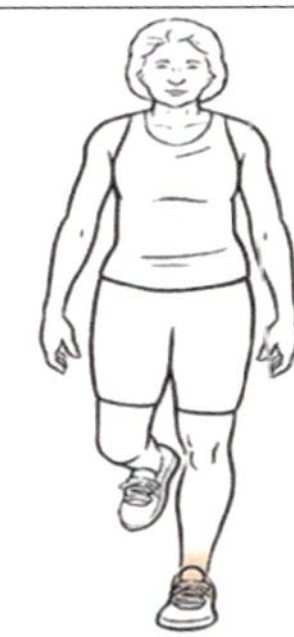
Sideways walking		**Heel-toe walking**

Aerobic exercises (5–30 minutes)		
Walking with rail support (low intensity: 40% of heart rate reserve)	**Leg cycling (low intensity) (40% of heart rate reserve)**	**Arm ergometry (low intensity) (30% of heart rate reserve)**
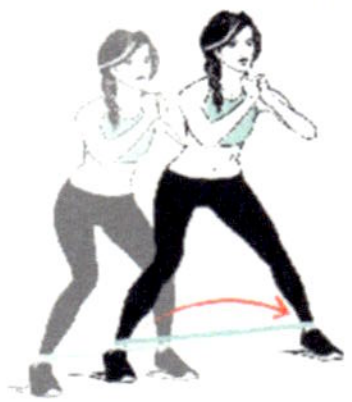		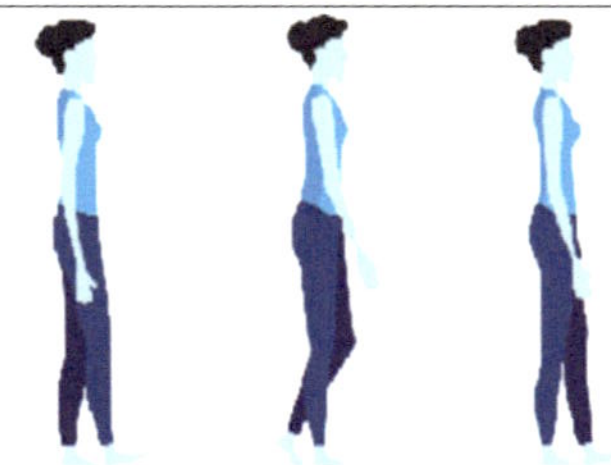

Adapted from Moore et al. 2016 [5].

Table 2.
Exercise rehabilitation programme for Parkinson's disease patients.

3. Conclusion

Empirical evidence has illustrated that regular physical activity and exercise may lessen the symptoms of PD and its risk. The evidence presented indicates that regular physical activity and exercise is a low-risk, financially inexpensive intervention which has proven to be beneficial to PD patients. Clinical studies have demonstrated the neurorestorative and neuroprotective influence of regular physical activity and exercise; however, more investigation is needed to validate the reliability of these findings. Medical practitioners should consider referring PD patients to clinical exercise physiologists, physiotherapists, and biokineticists to prescribed structured exercise therapeutic programmes. When recommending an exercise therapy programme the clinical exercise physiologists, physiotherapists, and biokineticists should consider the following factors: muscle atrophy (sarcopenia), muscle contractures, limited muscle strength and endurance, poor cardiorespiratory function, quick fatiguability, increased risk of falls, depression, and poor cognitive function which will impact physical performance and adherence. Careful planning will ensure a fun and enjoyable rehabilitative programme that will bring success to the PD patient.

Acknowledgements

The images displaying the exercises were taken from the Internet.

Conflict of interest

The authors declare no conflict of interest.

Author details

Terry Jeremy Ellapen*, Brink M. Ntjana, Chenelle Ribeiro-Wagener and Yvonne Paul
Faculty of Science, Department of Sport Rehabilitation and Dental Sciences, Tshwane University of Technology, Pretoria West, South Africa

*Address all correspondence to: tellapen1@yahoo.com

References

[1] World Health Organization (WHO). Ageing and Health. WHO; 2022. Available from: https://www.who.int/news-room/fact-sheets/detail/ageing-and-health [Accessed: May 1, 2024]

[2] Fernández-Argüelles EL, Rodríguez-Mansilla J, Antunez LE, Garrido-Ardila EM, Muñoz RP. Effects of dancing on the risk of falling related factors of healthy older adults: A systematic review. Archives of Gerontology and Geriatrics, 2015. 2015;**60**(1):1-8. DOI: 10.1016/j.archger.2014.10.003

[3] Giovannini S, Brau F, Galluzzo V, Santagada DA, Loreti C, Biscotti L, et al. Falls among older adults: Screening, identification, rehabilitation, and management. Applied Sciences. 2022;**12**(15):7934. DOI: 10.3390/app12157934

[4] DeTure MA, Dickson DW. The neuropathological diagnosis of Alzheimer's disease. Molecular Neurodegeneration. 2019;**14**:32. DOI: 10.1186/s13024-019-0333-5

[5] Moore GE, Durstine JL, Painter PL. ACSM's Exercise Management for Persons with Chronic Diseases and Disabilities. Champaign: Human Kinetics; 2016. pp. 273-280

[6] Sadowska M, Sarecka-Hujar B, Kopyta I. Cerebral palsy: Current opinions on definition, epidemiology, risk factors, classification and treatment options. Neuropsychiatric Disease and Treatment. 2020;**16**:1505-1518. DOI: 10.2147/NDT.S235165

[7] Kalia LV, Lang AE. Parkinson's disease. Lancet. 2015;**386**(9996):896-912. DOI: 10.1016/S0140-6736(14)61393-3

[8] Nussbaum RL, Ellis CE. Alzheimer's disease and Parkinson's disease. The New England Journal of Medicine. 2003;**348**(14):1356-1364. DOI: 10.1056/NEJM2003ra020003

[9] Kouli A, Torsney KM, Kuan WL. Chapter 1. Parkinson's disease: Etiology, neuropathology, and pathogenesis. In: Stoker TB, Greenland JC, editors. Parkinson's Disease: Pathogenesis and Clinical Aspects [Internet]. Brisbane (AU): Codon Publications; 2018. Available from: https://www.ncbi.nlm.nih.gov/books/NBK536722/

[10] Ridgel AL, Pollock BS. Parkinson Disease in Clinical Exercise Physiology: Exercise Management for Chronic Diseases and Special Populations. 5th ed. New York, United States of America: Human Kinetics; 2022

[11] Reich SG, Savitt JM. Parkinson's disease. The Medical Clinics of North America. 2019;**103**(2):337-350. DOI: 10.1016/j.mcna.2018.10.014, Epub 2018 Dec 3

[12] Bhalsing KS, Abbas MM, Tan LC. Role of physical activity in Parkinson's disease. Annals of Indian Academy of Neurology. 2018;**21**:242-249

[13] Papalia R, Torre G, Papalia G, Baums MH, Narbona P, Di Lazzaro V, et al. Frozen shoulder or shoulder stiffness from Parkinson disease? Musculoskeletal Surgery. 2019;**103**(2):115-119. DOI: 10.1007/s12306-018-0567-3. Epub 2018 Oct 1

[14] Rahimpour S, Gaztanaga W, Yadav AP, Chang SJ, Krucoff MO, Cajigas I, et al. Freezing of gait in Parkinson's disease: Invasive and noninvasive neuromodulation.

Neuromodulation. 2021;**24**(5):829-842. DOI: 10.1111/ner.13347. Epub 2020 Dec 26

[15] American College of Sports Medicine, Chodzko-Zajko WJ, Proctor DN, Fiatarone Singh MA, Minson CT, Nigg CR, et al. American College of Sports Medicine position stand. Exercise and physical activity for older adults. Medicine and Science in Sports and Exercise. 2009;**41**(7):1510-1530. DOI: 10.1249/MSS.0b013e3181a0c95c

[16] De Vos NJ, Na S, Ross DA, Stavrinos TM, Orr R, Fiatarone Singh MA. Optimal load for increasing muscle power during explosive resistance training in older adults. The Journals of Gerontology. Series A, Biological Sciences and Medical Sciences. 2005;**60**(5):638-647

[17] Katsiaras A, Newman AB, Kriska A, Brach J, Krishnaswami S, Feingold E, et al. Skeletal muscle fatigue, strength, and quality in the elderly: The health ABC study. Journal of Applied Physiology (Bethesda, MD: 1985). 2005;**99**(1):210-216. DOI: 10.1152/japplphysiol.01276.2004. Epub 2005 Feb 17

[18] Jansen J, Jollife CJ. Influence of physical activity on mortality in elderly with coronary artery disease. Medicine & Science in Sports & Exercise. 2006;**38**(3):418-427

[19] Braith RW, Stewart KJ. Resistance exercise training: Its role in the prevention of cardiovascular diseases. Circulation. 2006;**113**(22):2642-2650

[20] Verhaeghe J, Thomas JS, Van Bree R, Van Herck E, Bouillon R, Mosekilde I. Effects of exercise and dose on bone remodeling, bone mass, and biomechanical competence in spontaneously diabetic female rats. Bone. 2000;**27**(2):762-770

[21] Langhammer B, Bergland A, Rydwik E. The importance of physical activity exercise among older people. BioMed Research International. 2018;**2018**:7856823. DOI: 10.1155/2018/7856823

[22] Murray DK, Sacheli MA, Eng JJ, Stoessl AJ. The effects of exercise on cognition in Parkinson's disease: A systematic review. Translational Neurodegeneration. 2014;**3**:5. DOI: 10.1186/2047-9158-3-5

[23] Ahlskog JE. Does vigorous exercise have a neuroprotective effect in Parkinson disease? Neurology. 2011;**77**:288-294. DOI: 10.1212/WNL.0b013e318225ab66

[24] Kolk NM, King LA. Effects of exercise on mobility in people with Parkinson's disease. Movement Disorders. 2013;**28**:1587-1596. DOI: 10.1002/mds.25658

[25] Cholewa J, Boczarska-Jedynak M, Opala G. Influence of physiotherapy on severity of motor symptoms and quality of life in patients with Parkinson disease. Neurologia i Neurochirurgia Polska. 2013;**47**:256-262

[26] Kluding P, Quinn McGinnis P. Multidimensional exercise for people with Parkinson's disease: A case report. Physiotherapy Theory and Practice. 2006;**22**:153-162

[27] Allen NE, Moloney N, van Vliet V, Canning CG. The rationale for exercise in the management of pain in Parkinson's disease. Journal of Parkinson's Disease. 2015;**5**:229-239. DOI: 10.3233/JPD-140508

[28] Fayyaz M, Jaffery SS, Anwer F, Zil-E-Ali A, Anjum I. The effect of physical

activity in Parkinson's disease: A mini-review. Cureus. 2018;**10**(7):e2995. DOI: 10.7759/cureus.2995

[29] Scorza FA, Fiorini AC, Scorza CA, Finsterer J. Cardiac abnormalities in Parkinson's disease and parkinsonism. Journal of Clinical Neuroscience. 2018;**53**:1-5

[30] Espay AJ, LeWitt PA, Hauser RA, Merola A, Masellis M, Lang AE. Neurogenic orthostatic hypotension and supine hypertension in Parkinson's disease and related synucleinopathies: Prioritisation of treatment targets. Lancet Neurology. 2016;**15**:954-966

[31] Lang AE, Espay AJ. Disease modification in Parkinson's disease: Current approaches, challenges, and future considerations. Movement Disorders. 2018;**33**:660-677

[32] Shih IF, Starhof C, Lassen CF, Hansen J, Liew Z, Ritz B. Occupational and recreational physical activity and Parkinson's disease in Denmark. Scandinavian Journal of Work, Environment & Health. 2017;**43**:210-216

[33] Potashkin J, Huang X, Becker C, Chen H, Foltynie T, Marras C. Understanding the links between cardiovascular disease and Parkinson's disease. Movement Disorders. 2020;**35**(1):55-74. DOI: 10.1002/mds.27836

[34] Mak MK, Wong-Yu IS, Shen X, Chung CL. Long-term effects of exercise and physical therapy in people with Parkinson disease. Nature Reviews Neurology. 2017;**13**:689-703

[35] Real CC, Garcia PC, Britto LRG. Treadmill exercise prevents increase of neuroinflammation markers involved in the dopaminergic damage of the 6-OHDA Parkinson's disease model. Journal of Molecular Neuroscience. 2017;**63**:36-49